THE FIGHT

A H FitzSimons

Published 2015 by CompletelyNovel.com
ISBN 978-18491478-8-0

First published 2007 by Open Path Books
ISBN 978-09556111-1-7

www.extrememental combat.com

Cover: MICHAL BARAN

*For Nursing Sisters
Shonagh Jackson and Julie Christie*

Contents

Foreword

This foreword is contributed by Dr James Hawkins, a medical doctor and cognitive behavioural psychotherapist. In 1983 he was on the working party that founded the British Holistic Medical Association. He has written and lectured widely on mind-body connections for over thirty years – for both professional audiences and the general public.

The research studies, on which this foreword is based, are detailed more fully in the appendix at the end of the book.

This is the story of an extraordinary journey. Faced with an illness that became progressively more catastrophic, Anton fought against despair and apparent powerlessness. He overcame huge psychological and physical challenges. Against all medical expectation, he survived.

As a medical doctor with a particular interest in how the mind and body affect each other, I know such extraordinary outcomes do occur. However fairy tale endings like this are very rare. Are there ways that such "miraculous recoveries" can be made more common? I have great respect for good science and I think there are a number of position statements that can be made about this developing research field of mind-body connections.

Firstly, there is now overwhelming evidence that stress contributes to disease. It does this in several ways including through effects on hormones and the immune system. In 1975 Robert Ader and Nicholas Cohen published their ground-breaking paper showing that the immune system in rats could be 'conditioned' or trained somewhat as Pavlov had demonstrated for salivation in dogs many years before. This finding launched the field of psychoneuroimmunology –

the study of how psychology, neurology and immunology all interact. By 2001 a major review of the effects of stress and depression on immunity was able to report on over 180 study samples. Scientists continue to explore and publish more and more in this area. Many diseases can be worsened by high stress levels. This has been shown for cardiovascular problems, arthritis, osteoporosis, multiple sclerosis, HIV infection, dementia, type 2 diabetes, wound healing, ageing processes, some cancers, and a series of other diseases.

If a stressed mind can make the body ill, can a positive mind make the body well? The second position statement is that it is now clear that positive attitudes and positive support can definitely promote wellness. Coping style, a sense of control, relaxation and imagery, cognitive therapy, positive goals, and good social support have all, at times, been associated with encouraging changes in the hormonal and immune systems. An internal sense of control – knowing that outcomes can often be significantly affected by one's own responses – is particularly important. Unfortunately modern biomedicine may sometimes make illness sufferers feel that they are just helpless spectators. Patients can come to believe that the battle for health is being fought only by the doctors and that the sufferer's fate is entirely in the hands of others. Even the word 'patient' tends to emphasize this dependent spectator role.

The best supported benefits of a 'positive mind' and a positive approach to life are, of course, in preventing disease even happening. Healthy lifestyle is far more powerful than modern medicine in reducing our risk of illness. People who eat healthily, avoid being overweight, don't smoke, drink alcohol sensibly, and exercise regularly have only about a fifth the risk of heart attack and stroke of those who have a poor lifestyle. This is a huge effect, but only about 3% of the population follow all these common sense practices. Similarly research looking at 11 major types of cancer in Europe indicates that about 50% of cases could be avoided by living more healthily.

Can the benefits of a positive approach help once disease has become established? Yes – we know that after suffering a heart attack, being psychologically resilient rather than depressed more than halves one's risk of dying in the next 2 years. Similarly there is good evidence that risk of death is reduced by psychological resilience rather than depression following both stroke and cancer. An internal sense of control – that one is not just a helpless victim – is very important here. The link between feelings of powerlessness and depression has been known about for many years. More recently it has been shown that a positive problem-solving orientation is linked with a lowered risk of developing depression after major life events. Problem-solving approaches have been shown to improve quality of life in cancer sufferers. Reducing one's sense of powerlessness and improving mood also protects immune function. Problem-solving is an effective approach even when depression is established with a positive attitude towards tackling difficulties being particularly important.

Relaxation and imagery can also help here in a series of overlapping ways. Daily use of brief imagery focused on the challenges of the day and how to overcome them has been associated with greater achievement in a number of studies. Similarly, imagining and writing about positive experiences and best possible futures may produce prolonged increases in wellbeing and reductions in illness. Hypnosis and relaxation therapy can promote the immune system's health under conditions of stress. Meditation too has been shown to reduce stress while improving mood and sleep quality for people with cancer. It is not just a question of reducing stress levels though. Actively boosting positive emotional attitudes is likely to produce additional benefits for the immune system and for many other measures of physical wellbeing.

Not only positive attitudes, but also positive social support promotes wellness – and these two experiences mutually reinforce each other. An aspect of this support, which health care systems need to pay more attention to, is in helping disease sufferers realize that their own responses, wishes, and actions are all important contributions towards facing their situations as effectively as possible. Systematic review of the research shows that good social support approximately halves the risk of both development and progression of coronary heart disease. For men, this benefit appears to be, at least partly, due to a lowering of fibrinogen levels in the blood. Lower fibrinogen is associated with reduced mortality across a range of diseases. Research findings are less clear with cancer, but there is fascinating evidence that, in breast cancer sufferers, relationship satisfaction is associated with improved immune activity involving a substance called Tumour Necrosis Factor-alpha (TNF-alpha). TNF-alpha is associated both with tumour regression and increased survival time. Relationships affect our brains and our immune systems. Caring and love activate a rich network of brain pathways activating reward systems and quietening fear responses. Deliberately inducing feelings of care and compassion can boost immune function within minutes, while inducing a sense of frustration and anger can inhibit the immune system for hours. There is fascinating evidence that 'opening our hearts' in this sort of way – both for others and for ourselves – has important clinical implications, with pilot studies demonstrating benefit for mood and for chronic pain.

The third position statement, however, is that enthusiasts regularly make exaggerated claims for how commonly and how effectively we can encourage these positive mind-body connections. This is very understandable. It would be marvellous if we could all simply "think ourselves well". Very sadly it is clear that all too often we can struggle, pray, and try many different techniques with very little apparent benefit. Critics rightly point out that there is little hard evidence showing that acknowledged pathways linking mind and body can be regularly trained to produce important health benefits.

This is where reports such as Anton's can be so helpful. When territory is only poorly mapped, we need pathfinders to go out, explore and then share their experiences. This story is just such a report. Many pathfinders have been out to explore this frontier of mind-body medicine. Studies describing survivors of catastrophic disease situations find that there are a series of apparently different ways that people feel they have contributed to amazing recoveries. For example Warren Berland conducted in-depth interviews with 33 cancer sufferers who had lived for extended periods of time despite having been given a "terminal" medical diagnosis. When asked why they thought they had done so well, they rated spiritual, attitudinal, and behavioural factors as twice as important as conventional and alternative medical treatments. Berland concluded his study by stating *" ... the findings here clearly suggest that there is no 'right way' to heal. Some participants, the determined fighters, focused their attention on fighting to survive. Others prayed, visualized, changed their attitudes about themselves, and altered how they lived their lives. Still others believe their healing derived from a transformational shift that deepened their sense of meaning and purpose."*

Different individuals will continue to create their own pathways, their own responses to catastrophic illness. We know that these responses can hugely affect quality of life while living with disease. We don't yet know how much we can reverse illness processes. This is a frontier that is full of fascinating possibility. People who are currently facing life-threatening medical diagnoses, their doctors and research scientists all need reports like Anton's to help in developing improved understanding and better methods of responding both to cancer and to other diseases.

James Hawkins, Edinburgh, April 2007

Author's note

When I'm ill, I read to escape from reality. With this in mind, I have recounted only part of my story. However, this part contains key aspects which I hope will be helpful for many people also experiencing life-threatening illness. I have missed out a number of important factors: the support given to me by family and friends and my dependency on my consultant, not just for my morale, but for his unwavering stance in the face of medical opinion.

More than anything what's missing is the care, attention and affection bestowed on me by the nurses of the Surgical High Dependency Unit, Intensive Care Unit and Ward 24 at the Western General Hospital in Edinburgh. I was, quite literally, held together by them.

Part 1
Searching

I

The hall felt cold, damp and unfriendly as the man walked in. He noticed it had that familiar smell of bruised leather and stale sweat. It also had a familiar sound, emanating from the twenty-five or so youths, teenage boys mostly, who were either working on the bags, skipping or bandaging their hands. If youthful testosterone had a sound, then this was it. Clipped grunts of aggression fused into the jarring of limbs as leather pounded leather, as boys raced to become men in a high-ceilinged hall devoid of the niceties of a traditional gym – devoid of women, colour co-ordinated clothing, changing rooms, drinks machines, paper towel dispensers, air conditioning, any form of heating appliance but, most noticeably, a hall devoid of mirrors – for the youths that went to train there were not interested in how they looked. Narcissus would not be found in these halls.

The trainer was in his late forties, heavy set, his massive bare arms displaying tattoos including Para wings and his blood group. He looked curiously at the newcomer, sizing him up, knowing that at his weight sparring was going to be a problem. At this time the vast majority of boxing gyms in Scotland comprised of a selection of fighters weighing up to middleweight but not beyond and this gym was no exception.

The two talked for a while, then the man took off his jacket and hit the ropes, and his rhythm. He'd come to this gym in search of heavier opponents; the fact that there were none didn't mean he couldn't learn here. After thirty minutes or so the trainer called him over to work on the heavy bag. As the man bandaged his hands he glanced around at the testosterone sound system. It had quietened somewhat; there was apparently a growing interest in how he would fare against the heavy bag – an interest he shared himself because that would depend upon just how heavy it was.

He started up with a few simple combinations, loosening off his shoulders, getting the feel of the bag, how it reacted. The bag began to dance, swinging to and fro as he waltzed around it. He was the male, he led... *the very thought of you*... and in learning how it reacted he could continue to lead... *I forget to do*... and finish the dance with both of them in glorious, harmonious rhythm.

The sweat was running down the back of his neck now... *how slow*... in between his shoulder blades... *the moments go*... cascading off soaked eyebrows... '*till I'm near to you*... As he glided around the bag, he was oblivious to everything except the bag and the song that only he could hear.

The trainer knew he was holding back. There were a number of telltale signs: a lack of snap, hip movement, aggression. He knew he was holding back, he just didn't know how much.

'Last minute' the trainer shouted...

The noise that reverberated round the hall had never been heard there before. It was as if the bag itself had cried out in pain. The testosterone sound system blew a fuse and fell silent. Everyone looked over at the heavy bag that was shaking violently in some kind of unearthly spasm.

The man ripped out a second ferocious right hook into the lower section of the bag followed by a further three lefts, his left hip snapping forward with each one. Sweat flowed freely down his contorted face and with each punch he grunted out through his nose and clenched teeth, his sweat spraying over the bag. It wasn't pretty – gone were the polished combinations, the sharp footwork, now he just lumbered forwards and unleashed his power, his fury, and the bag continued its death throes...

In Hemingway's *The Old Man and The Sea* the old man looked back to when he was young to gain confidence in his fight against the great fish. The problem when I looked back wasn't just that I knew I was exaggerating but that I was beginning to wonder if it had actually been me. It was a memory from another lifetime.

After all, I thought, as I looked at my stick-like arms and the tubes going into them, *haven't I always been like this?*

II

The ceiling was my only place of sanctuary; everywhere else spoke of illness, discomfort, decay and depression. There were another five men in the room, most of them older. I didn't want to speak to them, I didn't want to talk about being ill, didn't want to hear them talk about being ill. I wanted to look out of the window at the sky and pretend I was somewhere else. But walking, even with the Zimmer, was a major event and the window at the end of the room seemed so far away.

My condition was advanced: my blood levels so poor I couldn't even commence the treatment the doctors favoured.

I'd been ill before but this was different. It felt as if there was an unseen force holding me down on my bed. The same force, having found its way inside me, drained me of all of my strength, not just physical strength, but as if it had torn the heart out of me. My levels of self-worth and confidence were falling daily. The feeling of discomfort that racked my body was constant and it was becoming increasingly difficult for me to stay positive. With the atmosphere in the room I was aware I was sinking into a state of depression; I knew that would suppress my immune system. I had to do something, anything, to break this fall.

I could do with a shower. It had been so long though, even longer since I'd had a cold one, and the thought of it exhausted me. I made the decision not to think about it; I'd go through the motions. If my body decided to stop me at some point, then it would do so, but I wasn't going to let my mind stop me.

I asked one of the nurses to disconnect and cap off my drips. Then, summoning all my courage, I stood up and made the long journey of about eight metres. I felt like throwing up by the time I stepped in under the warm water. I washed in slow motion and, when I was finished, braced myself and turned the lever from warm to cold. I was mentally prepared for this; it was something I felt I had to do to get the circulation going. I didn't think it would be that bad. It was routine, it had just been a while.

My bones turned to ice. I thought my heart had stopped beating and I was going to drop dead right there in the shower. *It's okay. It's just the initial shock* I told myself. But the longer it went on, the colder I seemed to get. My core temperature should have been rising, but wasn't. I stood there for several minutes leaning against the shower wall; somehow I managed to turn the water off.

As I dried myself I felt the blood flowing again, life slowly coming back into me, but I was shocked to catch a glimpse of another man in the shower room. I reasoned this man must have come in when I was numbed into semi-paralysis by the cold water. I was embarrassed for the man, about twenty years my senior, who looked like he was in the wrong place at the wrong time. I remembered seeing old footage of prisoners being released from concentration camps and this man's body was just like theirs: huge head; gaunt, haunted face; long narrow neck, supported by bones covered by an almost transparent layer of taut skin. The insides of this man's forearms and the backs of his hands were a mass of purple and blue bruises. I felt uncomfortable being in such close proximity to someone who was probably dying so I moved to leave. As I moved, so did the man. I turned and looked at the door I'd locked when I'd entered the room. I turned again and looked into the man's eyes. He looked straight back into mine.

III

What little there was left of my confidence and self-worth was almost extinguished. My illness took on a different form. I no longer saw it as 'life-threatening' but as something that was intent on killing me and was already halfway there. For the first time I was engulfed in a wave of fear.

I knew that fear could lead to despair. Depression was bad enough but despair was different. I had read about the devastating effect it could have on the immune system. My condition was so poor that if I let despair run riot I would die regardless of what the doctors did. I had to detach myself, look at things objectively.

My physical state had shocked me. That I was too ill to commence the favoured treatment was disturbing but the fact remained that I was still being treated and my consultant remained optimistic. So I had a chance. I fixed my eyes resolutely on the ceiling as if I could somehow penetrate it and see the sky. And escape.

There was no escape though; there was no way out of what was going on in my mind. It was natural to feel depression and fear but it felt like an enormous magnet was pulling me towards despair and I was powerless to stop it.

The hours of daylight passed as they always did in this room, the sun and sky never finding their way to my bed. The overhead lights were artificial, clinical, consuming in their depressive glare. Evening passed and there was just the humming of infusion machines, the distant voices of nurses carrying up the corridor. I used to love running at night. Now the night unleashed its demons.

The image in the mirror of the dying man kept flashing into my mind.

What are you going to do?

Fear and depression – they are trying to make you despair. Forget about the illness, that's not your problem. Fear and depression alone are trying to kill you. They've been trying this from the first day you were diagnosed. You just haven't realized it until now.

You're at war.

I went through my other enemies.

Every destructive emotion: anger, hate, bitterness, jealousy, self-pity, regret... the list just seemed to keep going. Then there was the pain and discomfort – those I had to endure. It was fear that I was most concerned about, there was no direct form to it and it seemed to smother everything, every thought. It permeated my entire being.

How do you kill fear? I asked myself, as again I tried to penetrate the ceiling and see the sky.

IV

Rose Street, Edinburgh; July 1983

Nine pm: As the man walked towards the club he rejoiced in the cool breeze and he soaked up all the sights and sounds of the summer night. He'd trained a few hours earlier and had had a cold shower just before he'd left his flat. He moved quickly, gracefully, in between the men and women on the pavement. There was an invisible energy to the night; everyone who was on the streets seemed to have it. The man could almost hear the night saying, 'Enjoy me now, for there won't always be nights like this. One day you'll be old...'

After greeting his two colleagues on the door, he moved downstairs to check out the bar. It was quiet and, although the music was loud from the giant speakers, the dance floor was empty. He cast his gaze over the bar at the barmaids who busied themselves not with work but catching up on gossip. In less than an hour there would be time only for customers shouting for drinks. In less than an hour this would be one of the busiest bars in the city.

He began ascending the stairs and he saw that the other two doormen were no longer standing at the sides of the door, as they had been five minutes before. They were in a defensive position, standing square on, blocking off as much of the entranceway as they could. In this way they made it impossible for anyone to enter without pushing or knocking them out of the way.

As he reached the top he was expecting to see a group of five or more young men. Instead he saw one older man, perhaps in his early thirties, tattoos covering his bare muscular arms. But it was the 'CUT HERE' tattoo with a broken line encircling his neck that summed up both him and the situation.

The tale of impending doom was unfolding when the man

gently pushed his shoulders in between those of his colleagues. Stepping down one step onto the pavement, he leaned against the wall and half stifled a yawn. It was important to have an open show of indifference when threats were made. It was important for the men he worked with to see his confidence. But it was mostly camouflage; of the three doormen he was probably the most afraid. All three knew this was much more than a threat. After a while of working on the door they had become attuned to the truth of statements such as these.

'There's twenty of us; we'll be coming in an hour or so... and we'll be coming in.' It was said with the smile of a man who knew that the three now facing him would either give way or be badly beaten for their naivety in trying to stop him.

There was no sarcastic retort, no 'We'll be waiting', just silence. The silence remained after the bearer of the message was out of sight.

The man looked up at the sky which had turned a dark orange.

Minutes dragged past, the night had suddenly lost its energy, its vibrancy, its joy. In their place were sighs: an air of acceptance. The man knew there were a number of things that just aren't done – locking the doors or contacting the police being just two of them. It seemed as if his two colleagues were just going to accept taking a beating.

He stepped back inside and looked around for something, anything that could be used as a weapon.

He saw it almost immediately, scarcely ten feet away from him – the makeshift cloakroom – a framework of iron: black, hard, heavy... unforgiving. It wouldn't be easy but the energy of the night had suddenly returned and it coursed through his veins. The iron would bend, and if something can be bent, it can be broken.

He didn't speak to the others, just calmly walked over to it, loosening off one of the supports from the main hanging bar. He sensed the other two watching him but they were silent; it was almost as if they didn't want to say anything that would break the spell, break the chain of events that was unfolding. He took the six-foot support and positioned it under the balustrade, feeling around for the right level of purchase. In the moment that he found it, he laid everything on it, his entire body, as if his very life depended on that one moment. And in that one moment, the moment when the iron gave a couple of inches, it happened.

The bubble of fear burst.

Tongues were loose, an outburst of relief as the other two joined him and for fifteen minutes they laboured. They then stood casually back on the door, their three-foot iron bars resting silently, menacingly behind them. They didn't care now if the group turned up, for now they each had a weapon to fight with; now they were no longer afraid.

V

There was only one thing I knew of that could lead me to a weapon in my fight against my illness – the placebo effect.

It was a huge subject that was still not fully understood. I remembered seeing the film *Anatomy of an Illness*. It was based on the true story of Norman Cousins, who had an incurable degenerative bone disease. For some reason, he thought massive doses of vitamin C would effect recovery. There was no evidence to suggest that this vitamin would have or did have any effect on his condition, yet he recovered. It appeared to be his expectation to recover that brought recovery about, the vitamin C effectively acting as a placebo, something tangible that he could believe in.

So, if I just believe in my recovery, if I expect to recover, this act will promote self-healing?

For your condition it's an unknown. But the spin-off effect of believing in recovery is positive. You will not be so depressed or afraid, you will protect your immune system from these destructive emotions.

How strong does my belief have to be?

The stronger, the better. The more you believe, the better your mood, the more your immune system will be boosted.

I remembered reading something about that, how feeling good promoted the release of endorphins in the body.

So, if I believe in recovery, then I will not only reduce the emotions of fear and depression that suppress the immune system, but I may actually boost it, and there's a chance I might promote self-healing?

A chance, yes, but at the very least you'll protect your immune system and allow your body to work with medication. It's fairly clear that the more you believe, the greater your chances of survival will be. The latter will increase in direct proportion to the former: the ultimate goal being acceptance of recovery.

So it's about finding a way to believe?

If you can find a way, then you'll have your weapon, then you'll be able to fight... then you won't be afraid.

VI

I didn't recognize any of the voices. I tried to open my eyes; they parted fractionally. I was looking through a letterbox, seeing only along the line of my body. There was sluggishness to my thoughts; I was aware my stomach felt like it was on fire. The nurses *how many were there – three, four?* were going through the process of turning me, changing the sheets. I heard my consultant's voice over my head, talking to the nurses, asking them not to move me too much. *Talk to me. I'm awake.* I tried to open my mouth but nothing happened.

The nurses were chatting away to each other... *don't they know I'm conscious?* They were talking about moving me up to the ward. At that point I realized where I was, out of theatre and in the recovery room. Then I heard one of the nurses' voices, 'there's blood on the sheets again', as she moved out of sight. Then they were turning me. *Don't move me too much. Didn't you hear my consultant? Why do the sheets have to be blood-free?*

Gentle hands turning, stomach on fire, over on my left side, clean sheet in, over on my right. I knew from the routine that they were almost finished *then let me go to the ward.* I heard the nurses' cries of frustration, saw red squirting over the nurses' hands, over the sheets. *I'm here. I can hear you. Please don't move me anymore.* I concentrated, tried desperately to speak, but it came out as moan.

Changed again, settled, now up to the ward. I'll be safe in the ward. My heart sank, the nurses' exclamations signalling that my blood had let loose again. *Don't move me again. Please let me go up to the ward – the sheets are clean, they're just red in places.*

I just couldn't understand why the nurses kept turning me. My consultant had clearly asked them not to. It seemed that if they kept turning me eventually the stitches would break or worse. I felt certain that I could summon the rage and adrenaline to cry out, to scream at them to stop, for what they were doing was madness. I considered it, but the effort would be immense. The strain of it would centre on my abdomen and probably burst whatever was on fire inside me. Even if it didn't, I feared they would just ignore me and carry on, caught up in protocol. *Then what would you do? Start fighting with them, grab their hands, beat them off? Then you would definitely rupture and burst.* I realized I had no choice and I forced myself to relax *just one more time.* Over on my left, over on my right, stomach on fire, finally on my back... *take me to the ward now, please.*

This time I saw the flash of red before I heard the nurses' cries.

I'm never going to get to the ward; I'm going to die right here. I'm going to die for the sake of white sheets.

VII

Ursula was dead. The mood in the camp was sombre, reflecting the loss of one of the ship's most valiant warriors. *Brave Ursula, beautiful Ursula* and I felt her passing more acutely than the rest of the crew. From my stretcher I looked across to where her athletic body lay, her purple combat suit contrasting with the planet's bright orange surface. She had been on point when the aliens had attacked and she had fought and died alone. I had desperately wanted to fight; I always wanted to fight, but I never had a weapon and was always incapable of getting up, I was always sick. And it was always the female members of the crew who were killed during these lightning attacks. It was always them that did all the fighting.

The voyage back to earth took several years: there were a thousand galaxies to negotiate first, crossings of time dimensions, 'holding stations' where we had to wait for galaxies to fall into alignment, refuelling planets and the sickness, always the sickness, always me that the others would make allowances for. When we finally returned to earth I found myself in a deserted restaurant somewhere near the harbour in Oban. But, as I lay in an empty room, I was still sick because of the space travel. All I knew was that I was going to be stuck in this room for a long time.

It was always torturously slow, surfacing from the dreams. Hours passed as I flickered in and out of consciousness, my hospital room taking the form of the room in the dream. When I finally surfaced from the ketamine and morphine I did not think about why I had dreamt of Oban. Nor did I wonder how much time had actually passed during the dream. Nor did I make the connection that it was almost exclusively female nurses fighting to keep me alive. I didn't think about any of the dreams when my conscious fully

19

surfaced. I couldn't, there were so many of them and they were so sapping mentally, so destructive, so real.

There had been a series of operations, starting with the removal of one organ and culminating in an emergency operation to remove a second. I'd been in isolation in the main ward of the Surgical High Dependency Unit for over two months. Bay 2 had become mine. It was a big room by hospital standards. Two huge windows flanked me, the one on my left looking out onto concrete and a sliver of sky, which saw neither the sun nor the moon. I missed a lot of things but I missed the sight of the moon most of all. The window on my right looked through to the main corridor and the nurses' station. There seemed to be so many different nurses looking after me, so many different faces; a blur of tenderness and caring. I was never able to remember any of their names, though I asked often enough. The sister was different. It wasn't just the navy of her dress or her being a little older, but her calmness, her grace.

For once my room was empty and I found myself looking at where the stapling began on my stomach. I couldn't turn to see where it ended so I counted the number of tubes that were going into and coming out of me. I stopped counting at seven; it was too depressing. Yet more depressing was my knowing that my blood levels still weren't good enough to commence the favoured treatment. Although my faith in my consultant was unwavering, my faith in myself, in my ability not to despair, was fading fast.

As long as you stay positive and believe in recovery, you have a chance.

How can I believe when I haven't started the treatment yet? How can I be positive when all that's happening is negative?

That was really the main issue: things just kept going wrong.

I was constantly plagued by an almost overpowering urge to despair. I was so ill now; I'd already been kept alive on artificial respiration for a week. There were voices inside my head telling me to accept that I was going to die and, as each day passed, they were getting louder. I met these voices with one phrase that I repeated over and over again.

The more you believe in recovery, the greater your chances of survival are.

The days and the pain seemed endless. Sometimes I would focus on a mark on the ceiling and effectively shut down, stop consciously thinking about anything. I just lay immobile whilst time seemed to stand still for me; it was as if there was no other world than that mark, nothing else existed. I would do this for long periods when the pain became too intense. If I hadn't, I would have despaired. I could cope with this level of pain but it was the relentlessness and the knowledge that there was no end in sight that I couldn't handle. It wasn't a case of there being no light at the end of the tunnel; there was no tunnel, there was nothing.

When the pain and discomfort lessened I would continue to try to believe in my recovery but it was too great a mental leap for me: too great a leap of faith.

I was now feeling the same level of frustration that I felt in my dreams; I wanted to fight for life in them but was never able to do so. The dividing line between dreams and reality didn't seem to exist anymore. I was in a permanent state of wanting to fight and of always looking in vain for someone to give me a weapon to fight with.

VIII

Midnight: As the man ran up the incline leading to the hill, the wind buffeted hard against him. He was glad he'd decided to leave his backpack behind. Of all of his pleasures this was perhaps his greatest – running on windy nights when the moon was full. With the backpack it was all about training, this was purely for the love of it. But he had to conquer the hill first. Though he'd done it so many times, it was never easy and tonight he would be going up it faster than he had ever done before.

All he could hear was the wind and his heavy boots thumping off the road as he ran past the infantry barracks. He'd be on it soon; he was fully warmed up now and he stepped up a gear, hitting the foot of the hill at a sprint. He was a third of the way up by the time the fronts of his thighs started to complain. 'Enough', they said. His breathing was still smooth though, his legs reaching out, cutting down the hill with each long stride. Half way up and he felt the pleasure of the wind across his face from his right. He looked straight ahead as the moon lit the white chalk of the rough path.

'Enough!' his quadriceps cried in expectation of what was to come. His boots slid as they fought for grip on the loose gravel, his calves voiced their displeasure, his legs, however, kept pumping away, yet he slowed as he always did: this final stretch was so steep, each stride covering a foot rather than a yard. 'Enough!' his legs yelled. But his lungs were yelling louder. The furnace in them was burning furiously, the fire from them stretching up and out of his mouth. *Just a little longer* he told himself. The wind changed direction and hit him full on the face; it seemed as if he was running on the spot. His thighs were lead, the furnace in his lungs now white hot. 'Enough! Enough! You're not going to make it!' *Just a little longer,* the voice in his head whispered, but doubt was taking over. 'You went too fast! You can't do it!' And the voice whispered back, *almost there, just one more second, just one more... one more...*

Then suddenly the hill levelled, momentum carrying him the next few yards. His lungs gulped in huge amounts of the night air. His steps were short and heavy; barely a jog.

His body still demanded that he stop but the promise of the run had him now. He turned to his left and as the ground dipped his stride increased in length. With the furnace in his lungs rapidly cooling he began to settle into the run. Now he felt the joy of it: hearing the sound from the tall trees on his right, bathed in moonlight they swayed and circled in the wind. He turned from them and looked ahead at the path the moon had laid out for him. His breathing smooth again, his legs light, his boots barely touching the earth as he accelerated along the skyline...

My conscious surfaced. The familiar hum of the drug infusions and vibrant colours on the monitor screens, coupled with the night-light let me know where I was. I was alone in far too familiar territory; I had been alone here for too many months now. I looked through the small gap under the curtain on my right to where the nurses' station was. I wanted to see the face of the nurse. Even if she didn't see me, I would, by seeing her face, be making some kind of contact. But all that was visible was the movement of her white uniform. Another world: she was fifteen feet away from me, but fifteen feet could as well have been a galaxy.

To be part of her world, where I could walk around freely, was a dream that no longer seemed possible.

What can I do? I have to fight off depression. I have to try to believe I will recover.

But something destructive had taken place over the past months.

24

I had forgotten. I'd forgotten what it felt like to be free of discomfort, to be free of pain. I couldn't remember or even imagine what it was I was actually fighting for. I was struggling to see images of myself when I was well. *After all, as I looked at the carnage around me, haven't I always been like this?*

I realized that all I'd been doing for the last few weeks had been holding off fear and despair. *But then I must be acutely depressed.* I couldn't tell; the months and the dreams were taking their toll. Nothing seemed to make sense anymore. I *knew* I should believe in recovery but now it seemed this was the only life I would lead. Recovery was no longer a figment of my wild imagination; recovery was an unrecognisable word. In the isolated world of my room I'd begun to feel that, in some way, this must be what I deserved.

I didn't even know what month it was – *June? July?*

For some reason I thought it was Sunday night: Sunday night, Monday morning. *Did Sister come in to see me last Monday morning?* A distant memory from years ago was registering on my conscious. I wasn't sure if she had, I just couldn't think that far back, but I found the possibility comforting even though I didn't really believe it. I thought about the way she held herself: her back straight, her quiet confidence, her every movement expressing total control, almost as if saying to me 'you will not die in my ward'.

There was movement from the white uniform: movement from the other galaxy. The pain in my back found its way through to every other part of my body and I searched for a reason as to why I was holding onto life – maybe because I'd been doing it for so long and, although the engine had stopped, there was still some momentum to carry me another few hours, another few days. I looked over at the curtains on my left. If only I could see the night sky, if only I could see the stars, see the moon. Then I thought about Sister's eyes. They were extraordinary; behind the blue fire that commanded respect from her nurses lay an unfathomable depth of understanding. My gaze would not leave them from the second she entered my room to the second she left.

More movement from the other galaxy...

The curtains on my left gradually lightened and eventually the lights on my right, in the corridor by the nurses' station, came on.

I suppose the impact was greater because I'd had a forlorn hope that she would come into my room that morning. But it wasn't just her warm smile, searching out and finding my eyes, or saying my name: it was the way she did it. Suddenly neither of us was middle-aged. I didn't just *remember* what it was like to be well, for two or three seconds I *was* well; I was young, I was fearless... I was indestructible.

Though her nurses fussed over me, none of them looked at me the way she did. The pain, the discomfort, was no less but something was different. She acted as if I was well, as if *nothing* was wrong. And in doing so it gave me a glimpse, not only into a past and forgotten world, but also a possible future world, an alternate reality where I'd already recovered.

As a result of this, some of my confidence returned and I saw things more clearly. I realized that I had failed to gain any real belief in recovery, failed to shake off depression. I had become frustrated because of my inability to fight. Although I'd identified that I should believe in my recovery, I still hadn't identified how I could think this way.

I now understood I wasn't just at war with fear, depression, despair, anger, frustration, in fact every natural emotion. I was at war with the thing that all these emotions came from, that they flowed from in a constant stream, beating down my will, smothering my every thought.

I was at war with reality.

For reality was pain. Reality was discomfort.

Reality was death.

How do you fight that?

IX

I was in the future, in a hospital somewhere in Japan. Everything was metal. My room was minute, the ceiling less than a foot above my head. The wall on my right side slid open and, still prostrate, I was slid out onto a conveyer belt. There were no nurses, no human life, just metal: clean and clinical. I felt terribly alone.

Pain reached me, cutting through the morphine, calling me out of my dream.

As usual, it took forever to surface. Slipping between moments of consciousness, I was transported to a number of different hospitals in Japan. I spent long days at airports, trying to communicate to the members of my family who were alongside me. Eventually I surfaced into my world: the world of my room. I saw the familiar web of tubes. I wanted to turn to my right and look out at the nurses' station but my head wouldn't move.

I had to banish the dream. To do so I had to distract my mind and think about something else. I had to create distance, a period of time when the memory of the dream would fade.

I stared at the fluorescent light and gradually the details on it became clear. I focused on one corner of it and wondered if the plastic rectangle there was a separate component. I decided it was and thought about the woman who had fitted it to the main body of the light casing. She had short brown hair and was wearing a green apron as she worked mechanically on a production line. I wondered what she'd been thinking when she assembled that part, her fingers touching it. I imagined her in the factory canteen during lunch, talking to her colleagues. I watched her walking home. She lived in a block of flats. She lived alone.

Focusing again on the corner of the light, I thought about the man who had fitted it into this room, how he'd opened that section to fit the fluorescent tube, his fingers touching the same spot the woman had touched, her fingerprints still there a year later. And if time didn't really exist, then on that piece of grey plastic his fingers had actually touched hers; their worlds had come together for a few seconds.

But only in my mind. Then I wondered if these two people had actually come together before in the mind of someone else that had lain in this room, thinking about anything, making up stories to fill in a few minutes when their minds were occupied: minutes when they would not let reality in, minutes when they would not despair.

After each dream I would make up another story. My room was filled with scores of men and women making things, painting things, and I explored each of their worlds, not thinking that they would never give a thought to the people who would stare at their handiwork and wonder about them for hours. I forgot each story; the drugs would take me. I didn't want to remember them anyway, for the people in my stories were always one dimensional: I never saw the wind touching that woman's hair, never saw her curves underneath her apron, never saw her smile.

My eyes were starved of beauty. It had been so long since I'd seen the sky, even from a window; it had been too many months since I'd seen tall trees bending in the wind, or felt that wind against my face. The only beauty I saw was in the faces of Sister and her nurses. I couldn't help staring at them whenever they came into my room. It was my one pleasure.

X

Although I'd clearly identified my enemy, things were no different; I still hadn't attained any level of faith in my recovery. As the weeks passed and my health continued to deteriorate, all I could do was endure. I managed this by holding onto a little scrap of hope that I might recover. That hope was all that kept me from despair. That, along with the drugs, the machines and the care, was all that was keeping me alive.

My sense of frustration had become increasingly acute. I kept trying to believe, but the act of believing just seemed impossible. The word 'unbelievable' in relation to my recovery had become cruelly ironic.

As I looked out at the roof of the hospital building opposite me and the sliver of sky, I wondered just how long I'd spent looking at this section of concrete. I didn't know what was inside this building. I'd thought about it often enough, though I had never thought about asking any of the nurses. Knowing wasn't going to change anything. It wasn't going to change the way I looked at it. That concrete was always going to be a part of my reality: the part that told me I was trapped in this room, the part that told me I wasn't ever going to see another building: for logic, my emotions and my instincts told me I could not survive.

It wasn't only that. Something else was happening. I could feel it growing in strength every hour. I was beginning not to care about whether or not I survived. Death began to gain an appeal in that the discomfort, pain and dreams would cease. It would also bring to an end my conflict with reality. I wanted to be at peace. Death would be a welcome release from the war that raged in my head. Everything seemed to point to it being the only way now: the only thing that could ever make any sense. I could see no future outside this room.

Up until now everything had been defensive. I had been holding off despair, enduring, trying to believe. It wasn't half-hearted; I was putting everything I had into it but my will had been breaking against a reality as hard and cold as the grey concrete outside.

A reality that was devoid of hope, a reality that said my life was over.

Part 2

Finding a Path

XI

I remembered seeing a film about a fight for survival called *The Edge*. The two main characters were lost in the wilderness and being stalked by a bear. The older man was bullying his younger friend into believing they could survive. He was referring to a book that described how a man killed a bear.

'It can be done. Do you believe it? ... then say it... what one man can do, another can do!' He screamed at his friend, getting him to repeat his words.

'Say it again!'

His friend repeated his words, this time with more determination.

'And again!' screamed the older man.

Finally the younger man screamed back, and you could see that he was actually starting to believe.

Yet when I said these words to myself they seemed empty and hollow. I thought again about Norman Cousins and his real life victory in *Anatomy of an Illness*. My illness was not incurable but I saw it as impossible for me to believe, no matter how many times I repeated the phrase.

But isn't that the key, knowing that the words will always seem empty and hollow until you start to believe?

Perhaps then, it becomes about fighting when there is no reason to fight, persevering until you reach the point where you do see a reason, where the possibility of survival starts to seem remotely feasible: fighting through the phase when there is no reason until you reach the point where there is.

Nietzsche believed that, with the proper *why*, a man can endure almost any *how*.

How can I fight without a reason? If I can't see any possibility of survival, why would I fight? This 'phase' is probably just a figment of my imagination.

XII

'You keep your eyes only on your home, blinded; you do not see that it is the journey itself which makes up your life.' From the film *The Odyssey*, Teiresias' words driving Odysseus forwards during his ten-year journey home.

In remembering those words now, I was driven to find my reason to fight.

Supposing there is actually one chance you could survive – it's there but you can't see it. Do you want to pass that chance by? You won't remember any of this, any of the pain or dreams when you're dead. There will be nothing. When you die there will be nothing. This is your last chance to fight. If you make the act of fighting your highest priority, you won't pass by the one possible chance of survival by.

You mean fighting for life?

No, if you fight for life then you are still going to be vulnerable to a reality that says you're going to die. Fight for the sake of fighting. In this case it so happens that you're fighting for your life, but it's the fighting that's relevant. If you can achieve this shift in priorities, then your fear of not fighting will become greater than your fear of death. Things going badly won't have the same destructive effect on you.

But how can I make the act of fighting more important than survival?

Reconditioning. Constantly reinforcing that you exist solely to fight and to fight to your best. It's not so unique; other cultures live by a code such as this. At different times in history – with the Spartans or Samurai this was a widely accepted approach.

I thought of a parallel where the focus centred on the commitment to 'the fight' – my grandmother's fight. My grandfather; gassed in the Great War was unable to work, leaving her with the task of feeding, clothing, and bringing up five children on the breadline in Glasgow in the 1920s and '30s. She didn't think in the long term, just committed herself on a daily basis to doing everything she could. I suppose she just accepted her life was a fight, a struggle, and got on with it.

Stop focusing on survival. Recondition yourself that the fight is your highest priority and commit yourself each day to giving everything you have. Paradoxically the by-product of this kind of commitment is that it will increase your chances of survival.

Perhaps it's possible. Perhaps I will be able to recondition myself but it will take time. How do I cope with the reality of death in the meantime, and what exactly am I going to fight with?

XIII

The film *Out of Africa* is based on a true story set around the time of the Great War. In one particular scene the subject of conversation was the Masai tribe, who had no understanding of tense, for them there was no future. They lived solely in the present. If they were put in prison, they died, for they just couldn't comprehend that there would come a time when they would be released.

Surely then, the opposite can exist, a person who can endure anything without depression or despair because they live solely in the future?

I didn't look at the parallel of how people were able to cope with adversity, a life of hardship, because they believed in life after death. I didn't look outside myself and my own fight.

The future, where you've recovered, could be your weapon. If you could find a way to think in the future, where your illness is no more, you would allow your body to work with medication. In theory it's clear; live in the future until the day comes when the future and present become one.

But how can I shut out the present: the pain, the natural emotions? How can I gain that level of control? With the reality that's around me, it's impossible to live in the future.

You don't know that. Too many things have gone wrong and you haven't started the treatment yet. If you think naturally you will either accept death or despair. Maybe you can think unnaturally by accepting that what you think will feel wrong. The only other way is to make a leap of faith. You've tried and you can't make that leap – your sense of reason won't let you – but perhaps you can inch your way to believing in recovery, work your way there.

I just can't think the same unnatural thoughts over and over. Can't you? Surely, this close to death, there are no rules – you can do what you want.

Even as a child it had seemed as if I'd always been allowed to do what I wanted. When I was eleven I spent the summer in the country. Up until that point my parents had just moved from town to town. I'd become used to moving, never staying long enough in one place to make friends. In some ways it was inevitable that I was going to become a loner: particularly after the summer of '69 when, during the long hot days, I went on adventures. Just after lunch I would set out, armed with a rucksack of food, in a different direction and walked for miles, arriving home only as it was starting to get dark.

In the spring of the following year we moved to the city. Then I went on adventures in my mind to break away from my hatred of school. In '72 I fell in love with Natasha from both Tolstoy's book and the BBC's television adaptation of War and Peace. Nights were my favourite time and, as opposed to sleeping on my bed, I took my quilt onto the uncomfortable floor so that I could stay awake a half hour longer in my fantasy world.

Remember how high your level of pretence was then. It was as if you had travelled back in time. If you managed to pretend to that level once, you can do it again. Make believe. Think like you did then; if you do it for long enough, it should take over. Ignore present reality and constantly visualize a future one where the illness is a thing of the past.

I had some idea of the mental discipline required. The task of staying positive for just one hour was daunting. The way things stood it was an impossible task. Yet I had the hope that eventually I might manage to convince myself that the fight was everything. Until then I would always be up against it.

Something, however, had been changing over the last few weeks. My sense of worth, which the illness had robbed me of, was returning. The nurses doted on me, but it was the attention I was getting from Sister that had the greatest effect. Every afternoon as she was leaving she called out goodbye to me. The first thing she did when she arrived on Monday mornings and the last thing she did before she left on Friday afternoons was to come in to talk to me. On Fridays there was a hint of sadness in her look, in her voice, in her eyes, contrasting to the warm smile she gave me when she returned to work on Mondays. I began to feel I was very special to her.

My self-worth and confidence soared.

With that confidence, when the drugs and dreams didn't have me, I furtively worked away in my mind to find a way to discipline and control my thoughts: to find a way to persevere, a way I could substitute future for present.

Years before I'd read about how the mind works like a computer and I determined that I wouldn't question what I visualized, what I programmed into it. I intended to ignore all negative feedback.

I would be thinking of a positive future but living in a negative present. There would be direct and constant conflict. I was going up against what I felt; if I believed I was going to recover, I would feel good. But the pain and discomfort were almost constant; the knowledge that things were getting worse just wouldn't go away. It seemed impossible for me to feel good. However, I reasoned I wouldn't start feeling good until my mind accepted this alternate reality. There would be a time lag until this happened, and until then everything would feel wrong, unnatural.

The time lag was the 'phase', the period when there would only be negative feedback, when there would appear to be no reason to fight.

But you've identified it. You know that everything will feel wrong and you may die in it, fighting seemingly without a reason. Remember it's the journey, the fight, that makes up your life.

With time lags, an invisible chance of survival, denial, pretence and fighting for the sake of fighting – I wondered whether or not I was just being naive. Yet I wanted to fight and these things were just a way of making sense of fighting when the only thing that really made sense was to accept that I was going to die.

I had to work things through and justify what I was doing. If I was going to fight, it had to be with total commitment. If I couldn't justify it, if I had an area of doubt in my strategy, then I would be beaten before I got started.

Perhaps the naivety comes in my estimation of my mental capabilities, of my ability to persevere. Is it possible to deny reality for months?

I looked at it hypothetically; if I were to recover then I would not have been naive. If I were to die without letting reality in, without despairing, I would not have been naive, because I would have stayed true to my path, true to my beliefs.

If I let reality in and died in despair then, yes, I would have been naive in overestimating my ability to persevere. Yet I refused to think that I was in any way being naive in adopting this strategy, for I could see no other way that I would still have a chance of survival, no other way I could fight.

In the understanding that, once I started on this path, there would be no adapting, no stopping, another issue was raised.

Though I had really nothing to leave behind, I thought about my relatives and what would happen if things didn't work to plan. I should really have made preparations before but I'd kept putting them off. Now I felt I had to make them.

I had a huge problem with this initially. If I believed I was going to recover there was no need to make any arrangements in case I died. I found a way around this by convincing myself it was to make my relatives feel better. Besides, as I looked at the giant window on my left, it was conceivable that I could be struck by lightning.

I didn't fuss over details; all necessary arrangements were made quickly. Once everything was completed I felt a sense of commitment. Now there should be no reason for me to come off my path, no reason for me to stop.

In theory.

I reminded myself that there would be no rules in this fight, but it didn't comfort me.

XIV

The psychologist sat on my left at the edge of the window. She was young and beautiful. She stared into my eyes waiting for me to answer her question.

She hasn't really asked a question though.

The long breaks in conversation were becoming increasingly uncomfortable. I wondered why she kept coming back when the meetings seemed pointless. I hadn't even considered explaining to her anything about my strategy. She didn't exist in my war zone and her prolonged eye contact was wasted on me. It merely made the eye contact I received from Sister and her nurses all the more meaningful.

Why does she persist in looking into my eyes?

I'd been immobile for so long that my level of awareness had heightened. With the psychologist I felt the eye contact was forced. She was just too serious. It was as if she was trying too hard. In contrast, the eye contact the nurses made was relaxed and came naturally. However, the nurses' priority was the day-to-day care; they had tasks to perform every time they came into my room. Consequently the eye contact they made with me was all too brief.

My need, my almost insatiable hunger for this contact, was only fulfilled when Sister came into my room. And unlike the nurses, she never looked at the monitors, drips or infusion machines. When she came into my room her eyes were mine.

I tried to work out what it was in her eyes when she looked at me that had such an impact. It was certainly something to do with the fact that she acted as if nothing was wrong. And that she looked at me the way some women used to look at me when I was young... and she had the most beautiful eyes I'd ever seen. But even so, I struggled to quantify how this simple act could have such a dramatic effect on my confidence.

I was aware that, in her fulfilling my need, I was becoming vulnerable. If the visits on Fridays and Mondays stopped, if she stopped calling out goodbye to me every time she left to go home, I would be devastated.

The near opposite was taking place with the psychologist, and after she left I told one of the nurses I didn't want her to visit me again. I knew that she was trying to help, but the fact remained she couldn't go into my mind, she couldn't turn off my natural thought process that told me I was going to die.

That wasn't her job. Her job was to help me find a way of coping with natural thoughts and emotions.

But I didn't want to cope with them. I wanted to eliminate them.

XV

I had begun to loathe the familiar glow of the monitors. I wanted the nights to end now. My sense of solitude was too intense during the night. At night I was alone and the impossibility of what I was trying to do was all the more apparent.

How can I continue to think of the future when it feels so wrong? How can I do that? It may be possible to do it for a while, but how can I keep it going indefinitely?

It was a question that I continually asked myself. While I searched for an answer the pain in my lower back intensified.

My spine was too straight. I'd always had to stretch it every time I trained in the gym. Now the gym was another lifetime, and the pain a constant reminder.

I looked out through the small gap in the curtains, I could see movement.

Come in, come into my world for a moment, just for one moment; forget your paperwork, forget the monitors and just sit with me and smile and tell me a story about your world, about your walk into work tonight, what the moon was like, about the trees you passed and the sound the leaves made as they rustled in the wind and how that wind felt against your face...

My tears were like unwelcome guests on a stormy night. It was a sign that my pretence was faltering. I needed to behave 'as if' I was going to recover and if I was going to recover there would be no reason for me to cry.

It was something that was happening more often now through the night: brief periods where I wept silently until I rallied and convinced myself that crying was a pointless exercise.

Sometimes it took too long. Then I would hear Brennan's uncompromising voice from the film *The Tall T*... 'Right now, you need a way to stay alive more than you need sympathy'.

But I didn't want sympathy. That was probably the reason I had reacted the way I had to the psychologist. What I wanted was someone to fight with me: to understand without me having to explain, just to play along in my game of pretence.

I seemed to forget, during the long nights, that this role was already being filled. Nor had I made the connection that the reason I wanted the nights to end now was because Sister only worked during the day.

As yet, I hadn't cried through the day. It was important to me that the nurses didn't see me cry, as if crying when I was alone was somehow allowed. The illness wasn't breaking me. I wasn't feeling self-pity.

That's what I kept telling myself.

XVI

One afternoon the nurses were sitting me up to move me to a chair and a reddish brown fluid started to leak through my dressings and onto the floor. Whilst I'd been lying flat I had been able to blind myself to the devastation that had taken place round my stomach: to the sheer amount of me that had been cut away. The fact that the wounds weren't healing was relatively minor when compared to this. It was not what I saw that concerned me but the image it represented, my life spilling onto the floor; I suddenly saw the hopelessness of my situation, just how ill I'd become and how ruined my body was.

I wanted to lie back down, curl up in a ball and wait for someone to come along and make everything better, for one of the nurses to tell me the nightmare was over. I wanted to be like everyone else who was walking around eating and drinking: everyone else that could go outside and see the sky, feel the wind, everyone else that could live life. I wanted to turn back the clock and live my life over again, somehow change things so that I wouldn't be here now. I desperately wanted to leave this room. But I knew I couldn't have any of those things, so I just stared at the small puddle forming on the floor.

As the tears began to fall, in the sudden awareness that Sister might walk in, I touched on a distant memory...

XVII

One am: It was two on two; there should have been no need for violence. Except that one of the two men who merely smiled when asked to leave the club could never be intimidated: the one that the man was standing three feet away from, the one to whom he was giving away five inches and fifty pounds, was a monster. The man had asked him politely for the third time to leave but was always answered with the same polite smile: a smile of confidence, a smile from someone who knows he's in control.

The man acknowledged that a level of violence was inevitable now. He didn't have to play out different scenarios in his mind. He knew from experience what would happen if he placed more pressure on the monster to leave. It would waken from its slumber and no longer be vulnerable. The opportunity existed to neutralize the threat, but the level of violence necessary was dictated by the menace of the monster opposite him... it had to be extreme.

Concealing his intentions wasn't difficult. The monster, so enclosed in his force field of physical superiority, wasn't looking. Even if he had been, he would not have seen it. The man asked again for him to leave, exactly the same way as the first time he asked, except this time he wasn't waiting for a reply. This time he was judging distances, calculating, sensing.

The opportunity he'd been waiting for presented itself when the monster lowered his head to talk quietly to his friend. The man immediately played out the move in his mind, the step forward, the slight bending of his knees, the downwards shift in his centre of gravity then the drive upwards, his head ramming into the monster's jaw. The instant he made contact in his mind, the move started. From being completely passive, in a fraction of a second he exploded in an act of unprovoked and seemingly unnecessary violence.

As I looked at my body again it seemed impossible that this had actually happened. Yet this time the memory gave me confidence because that monster was real, he had a name. He was well known in rugby circles, a touring international lock forward. With the back of his head crashing into the wall behind him it was his physical condition that had somehow allowed him to stay on his feet and half-stagger, half-run out of the club. An hour later he returned to speak to me and we shook hands. Then I saw the true calibre of the man and realized that had it been a fair fight he would have destroyed me. But there are no rules to fighting; I got the better of him because I had become the monster.

You can use this.

I saw the moment with distinct clarity. I had a choice; I could either let reality tear me apart and despair, struggle on and endure, or I could embrace it. An act of defiance was possible because I knew that death was close and my time in this room would probably be my last chance to do anything in life. At that moment I decided I wasn't going to let reality stop me from fighting.

My entire demeanour changed; the tears stopped as I turned my face to the nurses and smiled. It wasn't a smile of denial; it was the smile of a man who'd just regained a level of control over his emotions.

But it was much more than that. Suddenly I found myself acting 'as if' I was going to recover. In my calculated assault on the rugby player I had broken criminal law. In smiling now, and taking pleasure from an act of defiance against reality, I had broken something much more significant. I had broken a behavioural pattern I'd lived to all my life.

And something else happened. In one smile, one act, I had dramatically raised the level of my confidence and self-worth.

I knew about confidence in fights. Without it, you lose.

I saw it now; I had been programmed from childhood to respond a certain way to physical reality. When you're unwell, you feel bad physically, you naturally feel low. When things keep going against you, and it looks like you're going to die, you naturally respond with depression and fear.

Yet these natural feelings that go with adversity would reduce my chances of survival. They would stop me from fighting for my one chance. Whereas, if I acted in the opposite manner, if I could embrace adversity in this way the benefit would be twofold – I would be acting 'as if' I was going to recover and it would increase my confidence. The greater my confidence, the greater my potential to believe in recovery and the greater my chances of survival became.

Theory again. A few hours later my body was racked in pain and the nurses had to give me more morphine. Now I struggled to hold on. As I clenched my teeth to stop myself from crying out I could almost hear reality taunting me... try smiling now.

All I could do was endure. It crossed my mind that reality might be punishing me for my display of defiance.

What do you have to lose by embracing adversity, by continuing to act and think as if you're going to recover?

Nothing... so long as you never stop.

Don't look for positive feedback, don't look for a level of belief and just be content with programming the future.

It seemed that the only way I could persevere through the phase of constant negative feedback, the time lag, the period where there was no reason, no why... was to function as a machine.

If your mind works like a computer, are you not a machine already?

XVIII

Machine n. person who acts mechanically and without intelligence, or with unfailing regularity. (The Concise Oxford Dictionary, Seventh Edition)

In January 1977 the second squad to commence the first six weeks of basic infantry training at the Royal Military Police (RMP) Training Centre in Chichester was squad 7702. It was one of the smallest squads for this period, there being only nine of us. In the Army a soldier functions as a machine, carrying out orders to the letter. That was particularly evident in our five months of training. My friend, Jake, was injured and repeating a stage of his training with the next squad coming through. The other seven were, for a variety of reasons, unable or unwilling to make the transition and dropped out in the first three months.

At my first posting in Bulford I was attached to a NATO unit. Our platoon, of eighteen, the only one of its kind in the RMP, trained for exercises in NATO countries in Europe. The once a year highlight of this posting was a three month exercise in Norway. Our training for this exercise was the most physical in any RMP unit throughout the world. After a year of midnight runs, I was the fittest in this platoon, and, on paper, the RMP.

It didn't matter that it had been twenty-five years ago. It didn't matter that I no longer had the strength to lift a glass of water to my mouth or roll over onto my side.

What mattered was that I had once functioned very effectively as a machine. I just had to do it again, discipline my mind and shed all natural human emotions.

No, that isn't right. The machine you seek to function as is one that relentlessly programmes the future. Have you forgotten? If it hadn't been for your feelings for Sister you would have despaired long ago. You're being selective – attempting to crush negative emotions and heighten positive ones.

I then began to wonder if I had subconsciously chosen to fall in love with her: whether at some point an innate survival instinct within me had identified her as a weapon and selected the appropriate emotions.

I decided that was not the case. It just didn't seem possible that you could deliberately fall in love.

XIX

Why is there pain?

Minutes turned into hours and I remained unmoving. Pain was going to be my constant companion in the game I was about to play.

What is this place?

The drugs had me. I had absolutely no idea of what I was or where I was. I was like a baby who had no understanding, whose mind was empty, ready to experience and learn. When I surfaced like this I was effectively being re-born.

Among the first things I saw were the safety bars of the bed. I stared at them for countless minutes trying to work out what they were. I was trying to make sense, to understand. It was a natural reaction, to look around me for clues.

The dreams would give me a starting point. In the dreams I was almost always a sick man. So that was the first thing I usually became aware of. That part fitted in with the pain. Those two parts together made sense.

However sometimes, like this time, I began to surface and I didn't have a dream to give me a starting point.

My thought process was terribly slow as I sought signposts in my world of confusion. I would appear to grasp an understanding of what the bars a few inches from me were. Then I would lose this understanding because bars and any other objects couldn't make sense on their own. There had to be a framework for them to be part of.

Eventually I would understand that the objects in front of me were part of a puzzle. Then I would be in the heart of the game, the jigsaw puzzle that was my life. It ceased being a game when I'd put enough pieces together to make sense of who and where I was.

On the days when there was clarity, I reflected on what was happening when I surfaced from the drugs. I saw it as destructive. I was constantly being re-born into a world that told me I was going to die.

To counter it I had a routine that I fell into as soon as I was able.

Why are you here?

To fight.

Why fight when everything says you're going to die?

Because there might be a chance I will recover. I can't see it but I want to find out if that chance exists or not. The only way I can do that is if I exist solely to fight.

How are you going to fight?

By programming the future.

After a while the words no longer made sense, but going through the routine of saying them to myself was a positive act, I was actively doing something that broke the natural thought pattern.

Though I was working to control my thoughts, I couldn't control my body.

My stomach often went into spasm and I would vomit into the sick bowl at the side of my head. It didn't happen every time I threw up, but sometimes I would see the end of my feed line in the bowl. I was then faced with the knowledge that the nurses would have to go through the long process of re-inserting it, then, every few hours, drawing out from that line the mossy green bile that built up in my stomach. It had become normal life for me now. I didn't think about it, just as I didn't think about the fact that my urine and faeces had become mixed in one of the three tubes coming out of what was left of my intestines.

I didn't think about it because, if I had, I would have despaired. In my condition, I knew that if I despaired, I would die. This knowledge allowed me to use my basic survival instinct to directly influence my thought process.

Your body can stay in this room, in this reality, in the present; but if your mind stays you will die.

I turned my head to the right; through the window I looked at the nurses' station and the corridor leading up to it. I watched my future self walking in to visit Sister after I'd recovered.

But as usual it seemed impossible to identify with anyone healthy, anyone that could actually walk. I felt that if I could somehow personalize the image I might be able to identify with it. I had him dressed in my clothes but it wasn't enough.

Whenever I'd sent or given flowers to women it was always yellow or white roses. I couldn't remember when or why I started doing this but I began to favour yellow roses over white in the nineties after watching *The Age of Innocence* – Newland Archer anonymously sending yellow roses to Countess Olenska, and how after their meeting at the theatre he'd 'searched the city in vain for yellow roses'. It was as if these flowers had become a symbol of his love for her. With the image of myself walking into the ward carrying yellow roses for Sister I had a clear picture from the future of something that I could not only identify with, but symbolized how I felt and what I wanted to do.

Even so, only two seconds passed and the picture vanished.

I watched myself walking in again; after two seconds the picture vanished again.

I watched myself walking in; after one second the picture vanished.

The pain heightened.

Less than a second.

What seemed like hours would pass as I flashed images of myself walking in, never holding the image for more than two seconds. The images were always one-dimensional, always feeling wrong.

You knew it was going to be like this. Naturally you should feel bad, your mind should complain because you're hitting it with a false reality. When it doesn't complain, when you don't feel depressed, then you're in the future. It's about turning those few seconds into minutes, then into hours.

Remember, it's much more than denial; acceptance of a future reality is your weapon. You can't hold onto two opposing realities – the one that says you might die, you must let go of. Work towards accepting that you will recover. You've been through all the alternatives; this is the only way for you to fight, and the fight is the only thing that's important.

I would play out different versions of this argument, not only every time I surfaced from the drugs but every time I began to doubt.

My programming was sporadic. It was impossible for me to continually force unnatural thoughts through. For long periods I would stare at the ceiling and shut down. The instant I became aware that I'd started to think negative thoughts I would wrench myself back to programming, back into the future.

I began to gain some discipline in what I was doing. I was constantly policing my thoughts, checking on them, ensuring they didn't linger in the present.

Outside of despair, I identified four broad areas of thought. The present – reality – had varying degrees of depression; then there was the area where I shut down between present and future, the area of denial where my immune system would not be suppressed; then belief in recovery, where my immune system would be boosted; and finally what I deemed as my ultimate goal, the area where I accepted recovery and, hypothetically, my body would start to heal itself.

It was all irrelevant though. I was determined to programme the future, regardless. I'd worked out how I could increase my chances of survival and that meant several things – substitution of future for present, reprogramming of my prime objective that the fight was everything, embracing adversity and believing – something that I hoped would come naturally as a result of my programming.

Although I hadn't attained the level of control I'd wanted, my mood told me I was making some progress. Even though images of the future were still difficult to hold in my mind, I did not feel so depressed. There were brief periods of a few minutes where I felt optimistic. I understood that the better my mood, the more chance I had of surviving. It was, however, a difficult creed for me to realize. A re-education, a re-programming was required; the idea that I would be fighting by feeling good would have to be continually reinforced.

Each day I fought to become what I saw as the ideal, someone that lived in the future in his mind, totally unaffected by the reality of the present, effectively becoming a time machine. As I strove towards this impossible ideal, I pounded away at the heavy bag that was my mind, battering in more minutes of the future along with my new identity. And each day passed without me letting reality take over, without me despairing.

Each day I gained a little more momentum.

However, not all days were the same. Some days reality took its turn at pounding me, taking me to the edge of despair.

Part 3

Finding a Reason

XX

I surfaced from the morphine to find myself panting and with each breath there was a sharp pain in the left side of my chest. I was bathed in sweat, my back and left leg ached; there was nothing unusual in that, but the panting was new. As time passed, it worsened.

It was about six in the morning when it became clear that something was wrong. After one nurse had been in to look at me there was another, then another. My pulse was racing but the nurses couldn't understand why. I looked over at one of the monitors and saw the figure of two hundred; I was too busy panting two breaths a second to think much about this. My pulse had been high since I'd come into hospital anyway.

The pain in my back and leg worsened throughout the morning. However, it was the pain round my heart that I found hardest to bear. The doctors that had now appeared asked me to slow down my breathing but when I tried, even fractionally, it felt like a hot needle was piercing my heart. I had never felt pain around my heart before and, as the pain in my back and leg was now the worst it had ever been, I wasn't coping.

I looked out at the nurses' station. I was searching for navy amongst the whites and pastels. I felt I could stand the pain if I could just see Sister's face. When I saw she wasn't there I cut the thought from my mind, deciding it was better this way. I didn't want her to see me like this.

There were nurses and doctors surrounding me when my consultant came in and took my right hand in his. He then looked at the monitors and went over to ask one of the nurses to give me more morphine. I was relieved to see him but I desperately wanted him to hold my hand for longer. I still had absolute belief in him, as if by his presence alone, he could make the pain abate; but it worsened.

I didn't notice my consultant leave. Even though there were a number of doctors and nurses in my room, I felt very alone. I really thought about wanting to die. I could not bear this pain. I wanted to scream but I was unable to; I was unable to cry; I was unable to do anything other than pant two breaths a second and with each breath the burning hot needle pierced my heart. With each breath the vice around my left shin tightened. With each breath the invisible torturer plied his trade on my lower back.

Let this pain stop.

There was no respite. One of the auxiliary nurses sat next to me and held my hand in hers; I squeezed her hand with all my strength.

Two breaths a second.

A doctor who worked in intensive care told me they were going to put a line into my thigh. He explained that it would be painful.

The needle going into the major artery felt like a pinprick.

Over the past hour they'd identified what was wrong. There was a build-up of fluid round my heart and it would have to be drained out. The morphine must have started to kick in because, although my breathing didn't seem to have slowed, the pain had eased slightly. I no longer thought about wanting to die.

The doctor announced that I should be moved to the smaller high dependency ward alongside Intensive Care.

All I could think of was that, if I was moved, I would no longer get my visits on Friday afternoons and Monday mornings from Sister. I wanted to grab the doctor's arm and somehow let him know I wanted to stay in this ward. Then I realized I could use this. If I improved significantly, quickly, they would move me back to her ward.

I had scrambled around in my mind in an attempt to turn this into something positive. I could not, however, escape from the fact that I was going into a ward with the highest level of care.

I'd been in that ward three months previously, when the nurses had struggled to keep me breathing, keep me alive. It was a ward that had only four tiny rooms, only four patients. I hated that ward. When I'd left it, I'd vowed I would never return.

XXI

I didn't know the reason why but I had the ability to see through things. I was on an island with my wife and son. One day I was driving them in an amphibious red car across the water to the mainland. I knew my power of sight had increased and it was permanent. I was content in knowing I would always have my wife and son beside me. They were sitting in the back seat and I turned to look at them. They had no clothes, no skin, no eyes: they were just silent shapeless forms of red spots, red veins. In that second I knew I would be alone in a world without beauty.

Just at that moment a nurse came through the door. I opened my eyes, saw her in the same way and began screaming.

With the sudden surfacing from this dream, with the adrenaline that shot through me when the nurse came into my room, I didn't have time to get into my routine. My screaming had abruptly woken me and the dream could not be banished from my mind. It left me emotionally traumatized. It was pulling me to the reality of the present: the reality that told me I had no wife and no children. I was going to be leaving nothing behind.

You're going to die in this room, don't try to deny it anymore. There's no point. You're just delaying the inevitable. Let go; just let go.

I tried to find a reason to fight and start programming the future, but the present was all over me. Then I tried to shut down, find sanctuary in no-man's land. But there was none.

Despair was looming, hovering over my bed like one of the nine foot black armoured aliens from so many of my dreams.

There was no view from the window in this room but the door on my left looked out onto the corner of the nurses' station. I looked at this corner and tried to picture myself standing there. I didn't manage to hold the image, though I saw it flash there for a fraction of a second.

Initially I worked in what I thought were periods of around five seconds – every period I forced myself to see my future self standing at the edge of the nurses' station. I worked from one five-second period to the next, one minute to the next.

I knew there was no reason for me to continue flashing these images. I accepted I would eventually have to face reality. No matter what the doctors and nurses did, it seemed I must die. To think that I could recover and return to visit the nurses and stand at the nurses' station was impossible. Yet I kept flashing these images. I kept doing it because it was the *only* thing I could do. There was no intellect involved, it was just an instinctive act that kept me from despair. And as the five-second periods accumulated, the pressure on me to despair lessened and I found myself only having to flash the image once every thirty seconds or so.

My door always remained open and, with the nurses' station being lit at night, I was able to continue my mental vigil beside it.

XXII

Two weeks later I was back in Bay 2 in the main high dependency ward. I revelled in my reward – the twice-weekly visits from Sister.

Towards the end of that two-week period I grasped a greater understanding of what was happening. During the period when I surfaced from the drugs I was at my most vulnerable. This was when the war in my mind raged at its fullest and every time I had to fight the same battle to gain a foothold into the future. This was the point where my routine was crucial. Once I got into it, and had justified what I was doing, the rest of that period of consciousness was all about programming the future.

I fought each day to programme more than I had the day before. Each day I became more content in the knowledge that I was following the path I had chosen. Some days, though, the pain and discomfort were too great. Those days I endured – nothing else — and I felt fortunate to have been able to do so.

I was aware that summer had passed for the curtains in my room were closed for longer now. I didn't care that I saw less of the sliver of sky. Sometimes I felt I would have preferred if I didn't see it at all. It was such a small tantalising section, barely enough to be a reminder of what I was missing. Long ago, when I'd been able to sit up, the nurses had spent over half an hour getting me into a giant reclining wheelchair. One of the male nurses had taken me out of the main doors and along the side of the hospital.

My eyes had never become accustomed to the brightness of the sky, to the sunshine.

It was when I had been wheeled back into my room and they had started the long process of transporting me back to bed and reconnecting the drips that I had realized it had been a

71

mistake. I didn't want to see what I was missing, not when I had to come back to this room.

I vowed then that I would not go outside again until I'd recovered.

How long ago was that? How many months?

Time – how different it is now. How long a second of pain can be. How does it do that – how does pain change time, how does it alter time's fundamental structure?

When you're absorbed in something, hours pass like minutes, but with pain, minutes don't pass like hours; they become hours.

Rolling Thunder: one scene from this film had always stayed in my mind. The main character, an airforce major, was asked how he had coped with being tortured with a length of rope twice a day, for years. His arms behind his back, the rope had been wrapped round his wrists, his arms then pulled upwards towards the ceiling, until his shoulders began to crack.

The major explained he had learnt to love the rope.

I had tried to love the pain from my first day in hospital, but I wasn't having any success. I hated the pain, and a few weeks earlier it had got so bad I had thought about wanting to die. But I hadn't despaired. As soon as it subsided I simply went back to my routine.

The pain couldn't make me despair. That fuelled my self-worth and confidence. I'd already identified that the more confident I was, the more chance I had of survival.

Though I hated the pain, I had to admit it wasn't entirely destructive.

XXIII

When will there be an end to this conflict?

When you accept recovery or die.

Even if I accept recovery might I not still die?

Don't think that way. That's a natural way to think. If you accept recovery you will survive.

How can I know that?

I looked at my body. Apart from the massive internal damage a great deal of my stomach muscle had been removed. Yet despite that knowledge there was still part of me that longed for the life I used to have.

I turned my head and watched the nurses through the window and I found myself wondering about their lives. I was making comparisons and I saw how destructive this was.

You can't compare your world now to what it used to be, or compare it to any of the nurses' or doctors' worlds. Don't think about them. Their world is different.

I tried to think about the worlds where there were millions whose fight was much harder than mine, but it was too far removed. In my room I saw only people whose health appeared to be perfect.

Don't think about any other world. Think about the fight. Think about the future.

But what future?

Something sinister was happening today. A negative statement dashed every positive statement I made. I couldn't identify why I felt so low. As the day wore on I began to wonder if I had simply burnt out, in adhering to the routine for so long I was in a state of mental collapse. Maybe I had just given all I had. Today it really *felt* like it was time to stop.

I started to question what I was doing. I knew I was fighting for a chance of survival that I couldn't see. I knew my routine of justifying fighting and programming the future, made sense but I couldn't escape asking myself the question...

What's the point?

It brought to mind a conversation at the back of a courtroom involving the American detective, Kirwill, two of his colleagues and the Russian Investigator, Renko, in Martin Cruz Smith's Gorky Park. In answer to the question put to him by his colleagues 'What's the point?' as they vented their frustration at the system working against them, the irrepressible force of nature that was Kirwill, replied 'No point, that's the point'.

But today, I had to find a point to continuing, for today, I felt my journey was over.

What more can you do? Is it not time to stop? Isn't it time to just let go? Surely faced with continual negative feedback there comes a time when you have to stop.

Why? Because I'm conditioned to respond that way from childhood? Because logic and reason say so? Because it's basic common sense? Because of my human nature, my natural instincts, my natural thought process? What about my survival instinct, can I not just give that free reign and let it override everything else?

You've tried that and it's not working. Today it feels right to stop.

A couple of scenes later the conversation between Kirwill and Renko became an argument as Kirwill, in trying to achieve something his murdered brother had failed to do, said '... This way there's some point to Jimmy's having lived.'

Renko responded 'There's no point. He's dead.'

And there it was. In the apparent certainty that I was going to die – there was no point in continuing. Today fighting for the sake of fighting, for the one, invisible chance of survival... wasn't enough.

Today the machine had ground to a halt. I could see no reason to start it up again.

Kirwill, however, had been undeterred, in accepting Renko's statement he immediately went on to voice another reason to justify what he was doing. Instead of doing it for his dead brother he would do it for Renko. One reason had been cancelled out so Kirwill just found another one.

Is that the way it works? If that's the way then you just need to find another reason. You only have to justify it to yourself. You only have to find a reason that makes sense to you... why would you continue when it's almost certain that you're going to die?

You set out on a path knowing you would have almost constant negative feedback. You set out determined to do one thing – never stop.

I thought back to when I was in the Army and all my midnight runs up the hill. No matter how hard it had been, even with the backpack, I couldn't remember ever having stopped.

So what are you doing now – you're going to stop? Then all the times you ran up that hill were for nothing.

This time it doesn't matter if you make it to the top. All that matters is that you don't stop.

That you stay on your path, you never despair, you never give up on what you set out to do – that's the point.

But is it worth it? Is it really worth all this pain?

It wasn't the bullying or shame that worked. It was memories of the hill; the pain I endured to get to the top and the joy of the run in the moonlight afterwards, which allowed me to break free from the depression that now engulfed me. I'd found a parallel between the hill and Bay 2.

On the day I'd lost all momentum and questioned not just the point, but the worth of continuing I'd managed to start programming the future. I'd managed only because I'd realized it was late Friday morning.

Sister's visits on Monday mornings and Friday afternoons were brief, sometimes just two or three minutes. But today, those few minutes were the only thing that seemed to be worth the pain.

I had wondered before if people were able to endure a life of hardship because they believed in life after death. Now I thought about the millions who knew they would never recover, knew the pain would never leave them and I wondered if they endured solely for the moments in the day when they would be in the company of the ones they loved.

I didn't consider if I had become, or how close I was to becoming, one of those millions. All that mattered to me was that I had found another reason to start programming the future, another reason to continue the fight.

XXIV

My dreams varied: sometimes I was in field hospitals or concentration camps during different wars, sometimes I was in battleships, liners, lorries, coaches, cars. I was in so many different places in so many different countries. Outside of the alien dreams set in the future each dream was unique with its own complex story. In this dream I was in the present – I was alone, standing on a desk in a classroom of a school I did not recognise. My fall began in slow motion; an unseen force drawing me towards the varnished wooden floor. I felt a sense of relief in the knowledge that my head would hit the floor first, my frail body would be protected.

As my head impacted with the floor the crash I heard inside it far exceeded what I'd imagined. It was as if the floor was a detonator for the main explosion that followed.

Nurses all around me, hurling me round corridor corners, calling out to each other, as my trolley flew between the world of a fairground ride and an emergency scene from a hospital soap opera.

I was excited, caught up in the energy of what was happening, so many nurses, their concern verging on panic.

XXV

It was after I'd regained consciousness, when my speech and most of the movement on my left side had returned, that I saw my consultant. It was clear from the way he spoke that he was upset I had found out that the 'do not resuscitate' order had been given.

It had shaken me; I knew my blood pressure was so low I could have another stroke at any time yet, without really considering the implications, I'd made the decision to override the order.

My consultant voiced his concern about this information finding its way to me, about how hard it must be for me to cope with knowing my relatives had given this order.

I wasn't thinking about that though. I hadn't spoken since my consultant had come into my room because I was aware of an almost overwhelming need to plead to him not to let me die: as if, somehow, by showing to him my desire to live, in return he would be able to perform some feat of magic and make it so.

'Why?'

Silence.

My consultant looked and waited, unsure as to the root of my question, perhaps wondering just how much the stroke had affected me.

I blinked and waited; I was just as puzzled as he was.

More seconds passed.

'Why would I be upset?'

What is going on?

My mind was racing; I just couldn't understand why I was asking this question. Before I found an answer I started speaking again.

'It's in the past. I don't care. I don't care about the pain. I just want to fight.'

After my consultant left I stared at the ceiling for a long time, trying to work out what had just happened.

I had managed to put across to him that pain was not an issue but I'd also made a declaration. I had told him I wasn't going to give up. In its own way that was more binding than a banal promise; I respected the man so much I would find it almost impossible to let him down. In making the declaration, I was giving myself another reason to fight harder, another reason not to despair.

However, it was just as much a declaration to myself. I had been faced with a huge decision whether or not to turn around the DNR order. The stroke had been brain stem and the stroke doctors had told my relatives that, even if I didn't die, I would not come out of it, period. I had been lucky; I couldn't expect the same luck if I had another one. My open show of indifference was a throwback to a bygone age and I wasn't sure if I was trying to instil confidence in my consultant or myself.

I didn't think about the fact that there had been no conscious thought. I didn't see that what I was trying to create, someone who existed to fight, had perhaps, for the first time found his voice.

XXVI

The dream had been particularly distressing. Set in Burma during the Second World War. At one point the hospital I was in was being evacuated to escape from the invading Japanese. With the amount of equipment around my bed there was no way I could be moved so some of the nurses stayed behind to look after me. I was consumed with guilt that they were going to have to face enemy soldiers, and the horrors that that might entail, because of me.

When I surfaced I felt the same loss of worth that I'd felt in the dream, that all I was in life, and all I could ever be, was a burden to others.

I was so stunned by this sudden loss of self-worth that I didn't even consider the possibility that I might be seen as something other than a burden. This time I wasn't questioning the point in persevering, now I began to question my sense of self, my identity and the very fight itself.

You're a fraud.

I knew it to be true. I'd been pretending I could cope, that I could use the pain, that my confidence would increase and that my routine would somehow allow me to reach my goal – acceptance of recovery.

Stop pretending you're a character from a film. When you look back you only remember the fights you won, and they weren't fair fights. You always avoided fair fights. Why don't you remember the fights you lost? The most recent ones – remember the humiliation. Why do you keep pretending? Why pretend at all? This notion, that you can gain acceptance of something that's impossible to believe let alone accept, is just foolishness.

What's wrong with pretending? Does it matter? There are no rules to say I can't. What's wrong with doing it if it gives me a chance of survival?

The harm is in the despair and fear that will come when you stop the routine and finally accept reality, accept that you're going to die. Then the thoughts and emotions that you've suppressed will surface. You don't exist to fight and never will.

I thought about some of the men I knew from my time in the Army and from working the doors. Compared to them I knew nothing about fighting.

I'd had very few actual fights. As an amateur boxer, I failed. As a nightclub doorman, I went out of my way to avoid conflict. The only reason I was head doorman at one club was because of my ability to defuse situations. There had been hundreds of fights that I hadn't fought but should have: not only physical fights, challenges that I should have faced. Then I began to think about the other mistakes that I'd made in my life, the times I'd hurt people I'd loved. I had all these memories locked away in a vault in my mind.

Now I deliberately broke that vault open.

My life wasn't what I had done or had not done – my life was what I did now, today.

And every day I was getting a second chance. Every day I could erase mistakes and fight the fights I hadn't fought.

If I accepted I was going to recover, I would find redemption. I didn't have to survive. I just had to accept I would. By fighting for that acceptance, by taking on this challenge, I felt I could attain deliverance from my past.

XXVII

When the nurses' tasks involved moving me, I was not the best of patients. Every morning, when they had to turn me to wash my back and change the sheets, I cried out. It wasn't just because of the pain. Each time I was gently moved on my side, despite a nurse holding me, I was certain I was going to fall off the bed. With my lack of balance and the beginnings of bedsores, I resisted attempts to move me to a reclining chair. I'd been told it was important for me to sit up even for short periods in the day to keep my lungs clear, to avoid pneumonia.

I was at war with the nurses and physiotherapists on this. I felt I had to maximize my programming, not spend hours each day recovering my confidence after the trauma that occurred when I saw how desperate and depressing my physical condition was. That conflicted too much with the alternate reality that I was creating. I had to stay in the future, not the present. I found a middle ground, where the bed was inclined and I would sit as near upright as I could for short periods throughout the day.

I was at my most productive alone, when I lay flat, immobile, my eyes looking into the future. I never actually 'fell asleep', I was just knocked out by the drugs and my dreams continued to be endless and unforgiving. On the good days I would try to escape into another world, another universe, through films on television. Sometimes I would come close but the discomfort was always there, holding me to my world. I avoided downbeat films and I never watched the news.

I found comfort when the nurses would occasionally touch my arm, touch my hand, but there was no actual physical contact with Sister. I preferred this; it would have detracted from the contact that the relationship was almost entirely based on: our banal conversations ineffective camouflage for what was going on when she looked into my eyes. She was so experienced; she knew the isolation I was feeling. But she didn't know that her eyes had come to encapsulate and represent all that I was fighting for, all that was beautiful in life. In my world without a sky, my world of dreams where years would pass, my world of pain, the contrast was extreme, as was my dependence on her twice-weekly visits.

I wondered just how many of her male patients had gained comfort from the blue fire in those eyes. It seemed impossible to me that any man in her care wouldn't fall in love with her. I recognized too late where I was going with this line of thought, as logic hurled me to the realization that for scores of men, she would be their last love.

But I also realized that in falling in love with her, amidst the carnage of Bay 2, I had fallen in love with life again. If I hadn't fallen in love with life once more, I couldn't see how I would have been able to endure for all these months.

I again questioned the possibility that there had perhaps been something deliberate in my falling in love with her. Maybe the survival instinct worked that way. If it hadn't been her would I have found someone or something else to fall in love with?

XXVIII

It didn't come all at once. It wasn't simply a doctor coming in and telling me the treatment hadn't worked. It was more a slow, gentle process over a couple of days when several doctors came in with the same expression on their faces. They talked in the same way, the same tone of voice. None of them would look me in the eye. The scan results were ominous and everyone was waiting for the results of the biopsy.

It was a consultant covering for my own who broke the news. His voice was very tender as he said, almost in a whisper, 'It's not good news...'

'I don't want to die.' I regretted the words even before I'd finished the sentence. I could feel my chin trembling; the boy in me was saying *this isn't fair; this isn't right.*

There was the hum of the infusion machines, the noise of nurses walking past in the corridor; life was going on but it was on a completely different level. I withdrew into myself.

The afternoon and early evening passed in a blur. The closing of the curtains signalled reality closing in on me. I now began to think I had in fact been naive in thinking that I could persevere with a strategy based on denial.

I knew it was time to stop now, to just let go of life. Everyone had fought as hard as they could. Everything that could be done had been done. Yet with my routine I'd suppressed natural thoughts and emotions – I'd fuelled a false hope for months.

It wasn't just the realization that I would never get the chance to do any of the things I had wanted to do that hit me. My lack of religious beliefs and the knowledge that I had no children left me with one absolute and blinding truth; after I died there would be nothing. It would be as if I hadn't existed.

I had let life slip past me. I had not lived.

I felt despair suffocating me. I knew the risks I had taken in negating reality. Now, finally, I was going to pay the cost.

And that cost was high, too high. I had never imagined that despair could be so cruel, so terrible.

In a frenzy I scoured every corner of my mind, as if there was something I'd missed, another path that could save me from this torment.

Stop. Just stop. There is no other path. You know it.

No... I will not die this way. If there is no other path then I will just stay on the same path. What's wrong with doing that if it keeps me from despair?

Everything was based on the treatment working. It hasn't worked – it's over. You just can't pretend anymore, you can't act 'as if' anymore.

Why not? What's the harm in it if it stops me being afraid, if it stops me despairing?

It was all right to do when you had a chance of survival – you can't persevere indefinitely. You can't persevere until death.

You don't know that I can't. Think of it – a final act of defiance. A final act of pretence that would leave fear and despair vanquished.

But your pretence was based on having a chance of survival, albeit an invisible chance. With treatment failing it's clear that chance no longer exists. It would be madness to pretend you were going to survive now.

It was evident I could not survive, but I felt I could still win the fight, I could still find redemption. All I had to do was stay on my path and not let fear or despair take me.

The problem was that it appeared I had to be insane to do so.

XXIX

'It's a strange stubborn faith you keep... a sane man would have learnt to lose it long before this.' Quintas Arrius to Judah Ben-Hur from the film Ben Hur.

It was probably because my English teacher became animated that I remembered one particular class. Normally subdued, seemingly on the verge of falling asleep, my teacher's demeanour transformed when he described Hamlet's strategy. Caught up in an inexorable position, the Prince of Denmark wrestled in his mind to find a way out. His genius, as my teacher repeatedly stressed, was in his ability to convince himself and others he was insane. In so doing, it allowed him to escape from the emotional turmoil of the situation and secretly develop his plot of revenge against his enemies.

As the product of a line from a film and a thirty-year-old memory of my teacher's interpretation of a four hundred-year-old fictional play, I began to pretend to myself that I was insane.

This pretence opened my mind to the possibility that I could think whatever I wanted; so I could still pretend, I could still continue the fight.

But the fight itself had fundamentally changed.

Before I'd been fighting fear, depression and despair so as to allow my body to work with medication. Now I was fighting them purely to defeat them, to deny them victory.

What hadn't changed, however, was the way I fought them. But I found that as I began to programme the future it ceased being an exercise in defiance. I began to believe again that I did have a chance of survival, though with treatment failing this chance was now based on attaining my ultimate goal – acceptance of recovery, the point where, hypothetically, the body would start to heal itself.

Although I'd programmed the future and tried to think 'as if' I was going to recover, it was always an enormous effort to do so. I was still far away from accepting. It was this knowledge that gave me hope. There was no proof to say that such a high level of faith wouldn't, in combination with medication, bring about recovery.

As I looked across at the curtains on my right and the light coming from the nurses' station I realized that only a few hours had passed since being told the treatment had failed. In that few hours I'd known I was going to die but now I was back into my routine even more determined to gain total acceptance of recovery.

I wanted to understand what had just taken place. Regardless of the momentum I'd gained over the past months, I should have been devastated.

The film *Rashomon* is about an incident told from four different and contradictory points of view. The central characters' distortions, omissions and lies are not random, but strategic, given their individual situations, backgrounds and personalities. The way they perceive events questions the whole notion of truth.

My perception of the situation was extremely biased. I had always programmed the future in the hope that my blood levels would settle, that I would start the treatment the doctors favoured, and that it would be successful. I had, whether at a conscious or sub-conscious level, been selective in the way I coped on a daily basis with my deteriorating reality. However, with treatment failing, everything I'd been working towards had been wiped out. This news was not open to distortion; I could not perceive it as anything other than a hard truth. It was as if my levels of self-worth and confidence were so high I just wouldn't accept dying in despair.

In the early stages of my illness I had lost all my self-worth and confidence. I suppose that was to be expected, that would be normal. But, despite my health deteriorating, I'd managed to persevere with my routine and I'd begun to regain my sense of worth. Every week the nurses fussed over me, my sense of worth and confidence grew. But, right from the beginning, it had been the attention I was getting from Sister which had made the biggest difference. I doubted she knew just how effective she'd been.

Norman Mailer, a fan of boxing for over forty years, wrote in *The Fight* 'It was not unknown that a training camp was designed to manufacture one product – a fighter's ego.' It was unlikely Sister had read this. It was far more probable that she instinctively knew how important a patient's self-belief is, particularly when they are fighting for survival.

What a contrast my mind was to my ravaged, skeletal body. The scars – the hideous ones that criss-crossed my torso – were marks of my consultant's skill in cutting what he could of the illness, and ruined organs, out of me. Then I considered just how many times the doctors and nurses had charged my body with electricity to restart my heart after it had stopped beating. With the continuous re-birth process every time I surfaced from the drugs, I was beginning to wonder if I was just a product of the medical and nursing staff: an obscene creation, attached by tubes to machines which pumped fuel, fluids, oxygen, drugs, and every so often, blood into it.

But if they had created a monster, then perhaps a part of me was purely Sister's creation, for the man I had been would have despaired and died long ago. Maybe in all her years of nursing, she had learnt that, for a patient to be unafraid of the monster that ate away at their insides, they would have to become something ruthless themselves. Perhaps she knew that by looking at me the way she did and treating me as special, she would create a sense of worth so great that I could overcome the natural emotions of fear and despair.

I now knew what it was in her eyes when she looked at me that had such an impact. I had thought she looked at me the same way some women looked at me when I was young. I was wrong: no one had ever looked at me the way she did. She wasn't looking at the man I was now or used to be. She was looking at the man I wanted and needed to be, but never would be. She was looking at me as if I was the uncompromising Brennan, the unstoppable Kirwill, the cunning Odysseus...

And the point was that right now I really did need to be like these fictional, mythical men. Not just to have a chance at survival, but to stay on my path, to not despair. I needed to change, to become someone I wasn't. Sister looked at me as if I was a man who could persevere no matter what, someone who could stand any pain. Was it any wonder I was so dependent on her visits?

It was clear that the self-worth and confidence Sister had given me had a major part to play in the way I'd shrugged off despair. However I felt it wasn't the only reason.

I wondered if I had, after all, had some success in pounding the message that I existed to fight into a level deeper than my conscious.

I wasn't trying to override human nature; it had been natural for me to want to fight for survival. I was using that survival instinct to override my natural thought process, the way I'd been programmed to respond to my personal reality from childhood. I'd identified almost at the beginning that my natural thought process for the deteriorating reality I was faced with would lead to fear, depression and despair. Understanding what these emotions would do to my immune system had led me on the path that had brought me to this point.

It seemed it was the decision I'd made relatively early on – that I was going to fight and not stop fighting – that had influenced everything else. I began seeing things in a different way from how I would have had I not made this decision. I was seeing positives in a deteriorating reality purely because

I was committed to the fight. Had I not been seeing these positives, I would have been crushed by my physical state, by the dreams, by the pain.

However, being committed to the fight on its own wasn't enough. My ability to continue after being faced with the hard truth of the treatment failing was influenced by my sense of worth. With these two forces working in combination, I found that I wasn't just being selective as to what I now chose to see in reality; it appeared almost as if I was manipulating my reality, my identity, my purpose, so that I would continue reaching out for any chance of survival, however remote, that I might still have.

I was so caught up in the fight that I didn't notice the other force that also continued to reach out. The army of caring nurses that surrounded me, shielding me from despair.

Although a few of the doctors had quite openly shown that they felt all was lost, the army showed no signs whatsoever of giving up the fight.

XXX

Over the next days I stepped up the intensity and duration of my programming. For periods the future seemed to become my reality, even though this was in direct conflict with what was around me.

As I saw it, my conscious couldn't cope with two opposing realities. It wanted to accept one, reject the other, and put an end to the war. It wanted to accept the reality which it had been programmed to accept from childhood. It had always wanted to accept the present. It wanted to despair. That was the natural way. That would make sense. However, in holding to a strict routine, it seemed I'd overridden my natural thought process and gone beyond the point where reason, logic and basic common sense would normally have stopped me. By relentlessly programming the future, I was trying to force my mind into accepting that future. If I achieved that, then it would have to accept recovery.

It actually helped, considering my physical condition and what I was trying to achieve, to think of myself as a machine as opposed to a man. When I began to surface from the drugs, when the machine was switched on, it ran its start-up programme: identifying its purpose, its prime directive. Then the machine searched through its memory banks, ignoring anything that conflicted with this directive until it found the data that supported it, forcing itself into playing its main programme – images of the future – until it had used up its power supply, at which point it shut down. Some time later (whether that was minutes, hours or days, dependent on the drugs) the machine was switched on again.

That was the ideal. Even without the pain and discomfort it was an impossible ideal. Yet it was always a goal; it gave me something to aim at.

XXXI

It was the nine foot ones again: the ones that killed by touch alone, their thick black armour making them almost indestructible.

I was conscious: I could see the room around me but I was in the middle of a 'waking' ketamine dream where I was in the sick bay on a spaceship. The aliens I feared most of our enemies in the inter-galactic wars were about to board. I'd pleaded for hours with one of our crew, a male nurse, to give me a gun. I just couldn't understand why he wouldn't fulfil my request, why he kept lying to me, for I knew there was an armoury at the end of the corridor. Finally, in desperation, I asked for and was given a rolled up magazine. I held it fiercely in my right hand in the knowledge that, if I slackened my grip, even for a second, my weapon would unroll and become useless; leaving me unable to fight. I was convinced that my life depended on my grip and my eyes stayed fixed on the door, waiting for the aliens to enter.

As the morning wore on the drugs began to wear off and, though I still held onto the magazine, I became aware that I was in Bay 2 and not the farthest reaches of outer space.

Eventually I started wondering why I was brandishing a magazine and was nearing the point where I could safely relinquish my grip when Sister entered. She walked quietly up to the end of my bed and, looking as always directly into my eyes, said coldly, 'You're still having problems with those drugs.'

She had never spoken to me this way before; the usual warmth and smile were missing and for a moment I thought she was angry with me for beleaguering one of her nurses. Then I realized what was happening. She wasn't expecting a response, she was thinking out loud. I could see that she was certain I was immersed under a blanket of drugs and unable to see her. As she stood in silence looking at me, I became a

97

voyeur of what was going on in her mind. I saw in her beautiful eyes a sadness of such intensity I wondered how she could possibly bear it.

A full minute passed before she moved; then, shaking her head slowly in resignation, she turned and left.

As I watched her walk out into the corridor I was aware that no words past my lips, yet I heard them clearly, as something deep inside me called out to her.

I won't let you remember me this way.

It came as no surprise when I didn't get my visit that Friday afternoon or the following Monday. I'd seen her conflict: her compassion burning so brightly before being snuffed out by the acceptance that this was just the way things were. She could no longer pretend everything was all right. I had always felt she was aware how her visits affected my confidence and that, with the treatment failing, she would no longer want to encourage me. She didn't want to prolong my suffering. She wanted me to let go.

I didn't know that she'd stayed behind the evening I'd had my stroke and had sat with me whilst her nurses tried to get hold of my relatives. I didn't know the amount of death and suffering she had seen, but it was clear that, for one minute, a woman I really knew nothing about had come into the heart of my world: a world no one else had come close to entering.

I replayed her look of distress over and over in awe, knowing that no one had ever before looked into my eyes and, certain that I couldn't see them, shown their true emotions.

In my silent statement I was declaring that my love was powerful enough to be able to somehow travel forwards in time, walk back into the ward, and erase that look.

With my routine I'd been pounding away at reality. I could pretend I was insane but I was still bound within the parameters of my sanity, of logic. And logic was at the heart of the routine, always justifying why I should continue to programme the future, thereby continuing the fight. But logic had stopped me from believing, for logically there seemed no way that I could survive.

I may have existed to fight but, perhaps because of that, I had no real reason to live. The routine – justifying, programming – was a mechanical action; there was no passion. Sister had given me that; she had given me the reason to believe, the *why*. With her visits stopping, the only way for me to see her now was to recover. The only way for me to erase her look of distress was to recover.

The routine had been my weapon to negate a reality that told me I must despair. It had taken me to the point where I was ready to believe. Now it gave way to something that didn't need to negate reality because suddenly I found myself indifferent to reality.

I had, functioning as a machine, bludgeoned reality for months in an attempt to break a path into the future. Love had, in one minute, leapt there.

XXXII

Love is a symbol of eternity. It wipes out all sense of time, destroying all memory of a beginning and all fear of an end. (Author unknown)

It was different now, surfacing from the drugs. There was no gruelling routine to work my way through to gain a foothold into the future. I was already there.

In the afternoons it was as if I was fourteen again: the times when I didn't want to sleep. I lay with my eyes closed and listened on my personal stereo to my favourite songs and escaped into my future reality. I found myself feeling the emotions that went with doing all the things I wanted to do. I was planning and seeing them in detail: my eating and training campaign to restore my strength, visiting people I hadn't seen in years, walking in the wind, my reunion with the night sky and the moon that had lit my path on so many of my midnight runs. The list of things I was going to do kept getting longer. I didn't just feel the joy of being convinced it was going to happen; I felt immense fulfilment from the understanding that I was truly fighting for life. I had finally reached the point where I knew with certainty that I could do no more.

The rest of the time there seemed to be little or no conflict, even when the pain tore through me or when reality (in the form of the present) prodded me, letting me know it was still around. It was clear something had taken place at a deeper level. Perhaps the creed that I had found so difficult to grasp months before – that I would be fighting by feeling good – had finally been accepted. Perhaps the part of me that needed to accept the reality of the present had decided to stay quiet and let the survival part of me take over: almost as if my reasoning mind had grown weary of trying to force me to accept that I was going to die. In having warned me enough of the consequences of my actions, it had retired from its role as sentinel. I didn't consider the possible surfacing of suppressed emotions and terrible despair that would result if there came a time when I could not continue the fight. I didn't give it a second's thought because I no longer cared about any horrors or demons that might await me.

With love as my armour it was clear that my return to the ward would be the favourite part of my daydreams. The view was different; before I'd seen myself through the window. Now I saw the picture in front of me, as I walked down the corridor towards the lone figure in navy waiting at the nurses' station. I could feel the folds of the cellophane round the yellow roses I held in my right hand. As always, I focused on the blue fire in her eyes that was burning brightly again, lighting my way.

Epilogue

The story ends in September 2003 with Anton less than half his normal bodyweight receiving specialist treatment for pain from Palliative Care. Since his admission to hospital in February of that year he had undergone a series of major operations including the removal of his large intestine and a kidney. There were numerous complications including a blood clot on the lung, a brain stem stroke, and the 'do not resuscitate' order was given. Despite it being deemed medically impossible for him to survive, and under pressure from nursing staff to have him transferred to a hospice, his consultant continued to treat him.

He was told he was out of immediate danger in November. However having lain flat for so long it was to take over two months of work by physiotherapists to allow him to sit upright for five minutes without blacking out. The previous year had left him with nerve damage to his leg, paralysis to his foot, and osteoporosis. In March 2004 he was transferred to another hospital for intensive rehabilitation. By July he was walking with two sticks and was discharged into the care of district nurses and physiotherapists.

The following month he returned to visit the sister in charge of the surgical high dependency unit where he had spent five of his ten months in isolation. The meeting took place in the corridor by the nurses' station, during which the sister, unaware of the role she had played, told Anton she felt he should write a book about his experience. She was also unaware he had sent the yellow roses delivered to her earlier that day.

It was Anton's second visit to see her in May 2005, that he finally lived the image he'd seen countless times when he walked unassisted into the ward, carrying yellow roses.

The poem he wrote for her, *For Sister,* won second prize in an open poetry competition later that year.

Appendix

This appendix contains details of the research studies mentioned in the foreword.

The paragraph linking stress and disease is based on:

Ader, R. and N. Cohen (1975). "Behaviorally conditioned immunosuppression." Psychosom Med **37**(4): 333-40.

Zorrilla, E. P., L. Luborsky, et al. (2001). "The relationship of depression and stressors to immunological assays: a meta-analytic review." Brain Behav Immun **15**(3): 199-226.

Kiecolt-Glaser, J. K., L. McGuire, et al. (2002). "Psychoneuroimmunology: psychological influences on immune function and health." J Consult Clin Psychol **70**(3): 537-47.

The next paragraph introducing benefits from a 'positive mind' mentions research findings from:

Stowell, J. R., J. K. Kiecolt-Glaser, et al. (2001). "Perceived stress and cellular immunity: when coping counts." J Behav Med **24**(4): 323-39.

Sturmer, T., P. Hasselbach, et al. (2006). "Personality, lifestyle, and risk of cardiovascular disease and cancer: follow-up of population based cohort." BMJ **332**: 1359-65.

Comments about healthy lifestyle and disease prevention are based on:

Stampfer, M. J., F. B. Hu, et al. (2000). "Primary prevention of coronary heart disease in women through diet and lifestyle." N Engl J Med **343**(1): 16-22.

Reeves, M. J. and A. P. Rafferty (2005). "Healthy lifestyle characteristics among adults in the United States, 2000." Arch Intern Med **165**(8): 854-7.

Soerjomataram, I., E. de Vries, et al. (2006). "Excess of cancers in Europe: A study of eleven major cancers amenable to lifestyle change." International Journal of Cancer **120**(6): 1336-43.

The paragraph on the benefits of a positive approach even when disease has become established mentions:

Barth, J., M. Schumacher, et al. (2004). "Depression as a risk factor for mortality in patients with coronary heart disease: a meta-analysis." Psychosom Med **66**(6): 802-13.

Williams, L. S., S. S. Ghose, et al. (2004). "Depression and Other Mental Health Diagnoses Increase Mortality Risk After Ischemic Stroke." Am J Psychiatry **161**(6): 1090-1095.

Brown, K. W., A. R. Levy, et al. (2003). "Psychological distress and cancer survival: a follow-up 10 years after diagnosis." Psychosom Med **65**(4): 636-43.

Beresford, T. P., J. Alfers, et al. (2006). "Cancer Survival Probability as a Function of Ego Defense (Adaptive) Mechanisms Versus Depressive Symptoms." Psychosomatics **47**(3): 247-253.

Benassi, V. A., P. D. Sweeney, et al. (1988). "Is there a relation between locus of control orientation and depression?" J Abnorm Psychol **97**(3): 357-67.

Spence, S. H., J. Sheffield, et al. (2002). "Problem-solving orientation and attributional style: moderators of the impact of negative life events on the development of depressive symptoms in adolescence?" J Clin Child Adolesc Psychol **31**(2): 219-29.

Nezu, A. M., C. M. Nezu, et al. (2003). "Project Genesis: assessing the efficacy of problem-solving therapy for distressed adult cancer patients." J Consult Clin Psychol **71**(6): 1036-48.

Reynaert, C., P. Janne, et al. (1995). "From health locus of control to immune control: internal locus of control has a buffering effect on natural killer cell activity decrease in major depression." Acta Psychiatr Scand **92**(4): 294-300.

Cruess, D. G., S. D. Douglas, et al. (2005). "Association of resolution of major depression with increased natural killer cell activity among HIV-seropositive women." Am J Psychiatry **162**(11): 2125-30.

Cuijpers, P., A. van Straten, et al. (2006). "Problem solving therapies for depression: A meta-analysis." Eur Psychiatry.

Nezu, A. M. and M. G. Perri (1989). "Social problem-solving therapy for unipolar depression: an initial dismantling investigation." J Consult Clin Psychol **57**(3): 408-13.

The section on relaxation, imagery and positive emotion is from:

Taylor, S. E., L. B. Pham, et al. (1998). "Harnessing the imagination. Mental simulation, self-regulation, and coping." Am Psychol **53**(4): 429-39.

King, L. A. (2001). "The Health Benefits of Writing about Life Goals." Pers Soc Psychol Bull **27**(7): 798-807.

Burton, C. M. and L. A. King (2004). "The health benefits of writing about intensely positive experiences." Journal of Research in Personality **38**(2): 150-163.

Kiecolt-Glaser, J. K., P. T. Marucha, et al. (2001). "Hypnosis as a modulator of cellular immune dysregulation during acute stress." J Consult Clin Psychol **69**(4): 674-82.

Smith, J. E., J. Richardson, et al. (2005). "Mindfulness-Based Stress Reduction as supportive therapy in cancer care: systematic review." J Adv Nurs **52**(3): 315-27.

Kiecolt-Glaser, J. K. and R. Glaser (1999). "Psychoneuroimmunology and cancer: fact or fiction?" Eur J Cancer **35**(11): 1603-7.

Kiecolt-Glaser, J. K., L. McGuire, et al. (2002). "Emotions, morbidity, and mortality: new perspectives from psychoneuroimmunology." <u>Annu Rev Psychol</u> **53**: 83-107.

Glaser, R. and J. K. Kiecolt-Glaser (2005). "Stress-induced immune dysfunction: implications for health." <u>Nat Rev Immunol</u> **5**(3): 243-51.

Cohen, S., C. M. Alper, et al. (2006). "Positive emotional style predicts resistance to illness after experimental exposure to rhinovirus or influenza a virus." <u>Psychosom Med</u> **68**(6): 809-15.

Ryff, C. D., G. Dienberg Love, et al. (2006). "Psychological well-being and ill-being: do they have distinct or mirrored biological correlates?" <u>Psychother Psychosom</u> **75**(2): 85-95.

The paragraph on social support and the effects of caring and compassion refers to:

Ryan, R. M., J. Kuhl, et al. (1997). "Nature and autonomy: an organizational view of social and neurobiological aspects of self-regulation in behavior and development." <u>Dev Psychopathol</u> **9**(4): 701-28.

Ryan, R. M. and E. L. Deci (2000). "Self-determination theory and the facilitation of intrinsic motivation, social development, and well-being." <u>Am Psychol</u> **55**(1): 68-78.

Williams, G. C., H. A. McGregor, et al. (2006). "Testing a self-determination theory intervention for motivating tobacco cessation: supporting autonomy and competence in a clinical trial." <u>Health Psychol</u> **25**(1): 91-101.

Lett, H. S., J. A. Blumenthal, et al. (2005). "Social Support and Coronary Heart Disease: Epidemiologic Evidence and Implications for Treatment." <u>Psychosom Med</u> **67**(6): 869-878.

Loucks, E. B., L. F. Berkman, et al. (2005). "Social integration is associated with fibrinogen concentration in elderly men." <u>Psychosom Med</u> **67**(3): 353-8.

Fibrinogen Studies, C. (2005). "Plasma Fibrinogen Level and the Risk of Major Cardiovascular Diseases and Nonvascular Mortality: An Individual Participant Meta-analysis." <u>JAMA</u> **294**(14): 1799-1809.

Marucha, P. T., T. R. Crespin, et al. (2005). "TNF-alpha levels in cancer patients relate to social variables." <u>Brain Behav Immun</u> **19**(6): 521-5.

Bartels, A. and S. Zeki (2004). "The neural correlates of maternal and romantic love." <u>Neuroimage</u> **21**(3): 1155-66.

Debiec, J. (2005). "Peptides of love and fear: vasopressin and oxytocin modulate the integration of information in the amygdala." <u>Bioessays</u> **27**(9): 869-73.

Rein, G. and e. al. (1995). "The physiological and psychological effects of compassion and anger." <u>J Adv Med</u> **8**: 87-105.

Gilbert, P. and C. Irons (2004). "A pilot exploration of the use of compassionate images in a group of self-critical people." <u>Memory</u> **12**(4): 507-16.

Carson, J. W., F. J. Keefe, et al. (2005). "Loving-kindness meditation for chronic low back pain: results from a pilot trial." <u>J Holist Nurs</u> **23**(3): 287-304.

The comments about exaggerated claims and the findings on the different ways that people feel they have contributed to amazing recoveries can be found in:

Petticrew, M., R. Bell, et al. (2002). "Influence of psychological coping on survival and recurrence in people with cancer: systematic review." BMJ 325(7372): 1066-.

Sampson, W. (2002). "Controversies in cancer and the mind: effects of psychosocial support." Semin Oncol 29(6): 595-600.

Berland, W. (1995). "Unexpected cancer recovery: why patients believe they survive." Advances: The Journal of Mind-Body Health 11(4): 5-19.

Copyright Acknowledgements/References

The Old Man and the Sea by Ernest Hemingway Copyright 1952 published by Charles Scribner's Sons

The Very Thought of You by Ray Noble Copyright 1934

Anatomy of an Illness 1984 produced by CBS Entertainment Production, Hamner Productions Inc, Jerry Gershwin Productions

The Edge 1997 produced by Twentieth Century Fox, Art Linson Productions

The Odyssey 1997 produced by American Zoetrope, Beta Film GmbH, Hallmark Entertainment, KirchMedia, Mediaset, ProSieben Media AG, Remote Camera Systems, Skai TV

War and Peace by Leo Tolstoy 1869 produced for the BBC by David Conroy 1972

Out of Africa 1985 produced by Universal Pictures, Mirage Entertainment

The Tall T 1957 produced by Columbia Pictures Corporation, Producers-Actors Corporation

The Age Of Innocence 1993 produced by Columbia Pictures Corporation, Cappa Production

Rolling Thunder 1977 produced by American International Pictures

Gorky Park by Martin Cruz Smith Copyright 1981 published by Random House & GK Hall

Rashomon 1950 produced by Daiei Motion Picture Co. Ltd, Daiei Studios

Acknowledgments

I thank Dr James Hawkins, Freya Ferguson, James Lindsay, Robert McCall, Dugald McCallum, and Debbie Middleton for their generous aid and encouragement during the writing of this book. My thanks also to the printers Wm. Anderson & Sons Ltd, Glasgow.

Also by A H FitzSimons

Non-fiction

EXTREME MENTAL COMBAT

Fiction

THE GAME

BREAK LIMA